To Trish,

I hope you enjoy this trip into the future,

best wishes

[illegible]

RIYADH

14/1/96.

Beyond the Barrier

Beyond the Barrier

Graham Miller

The Book Guild Ltd.
Sussex, England

To my parents

Thelma and Lindsay Miller

This book is a work of fiction. The characters and situations in this story are imaginary. No resemblence is intended between these characters and any real persons, either living or dead.

The Book Guild Ltd.
25 High Street,
Lewes, Sussex

First published 1993

Set in Baskerville
Typesetting by Ashford Setting and Design Services
Ashford, Middlesex
Printed in Great Britain by
Antony Rowe Ltd.
Chippenham, Wiltshire.

A catalogue record for this book is available
from the British Library

ISBN 0 86332 888 1

1

2030

Unravel the greatest mystery of the twenty first century? It seemed a highly unlikely possibility on this blustery overcast night. It certainly was not amongst Ben Andrew's wildest dreams as he jogged towards the communications building. Ben had other things on his mind. A creature of habit, he rarely ran late. In fact it was at least half an hour before his shift began. Yet he muttered to himself whilst repeatedly peering at his watch, hoping perhaps it might freeze or even reverse its relentless forward motion. On arrival at the entrance to the building, he blustered uncharacteristically at the security guard: 'Max! . . . has a young man arrived? I had hoped to be here before him. I'll bet I'm late. No points for manners for me tonight . . .'

Ben's torrent of words was hardly intelligible, yet Max grasped the essentials of the outburst and replied soothingly, 'No need to worry, Ben, he's already here. I've welcomed him to our illustrious institution, shown him around and . . . even given him a cup of our infamous coffee. That's him over there.'

Ben's eyes flashed across the foyer. Having sped across the open ground from the car park, he now stood motionless in the doorway, allowing an unpleasant draught to enter.

Max tactfully eased Ben inside and closed the door. Ben then recommenced his headlong rush, his shoes clicking and scraping across the tiled floor. His quarry was propped against a reception desk. So determined was Ben to make contact that he barely noticed a pretty young woman with a shock of striking blonde hair. She turned slightly in response to the clatter of Ben's approach, then appeared to duck her head as she caught sight of him. In spite of her attractiveness, Ben's attention remained steadfastly attached to the young man whom he addressed as he approached.

'Peter! Peter Spence?'

'That's me,' replied the young man.

'I'm dreadfully sorry, I'd planned to arrive before you and welcome you.'

'No problem,' interrupted Peter. 'Max, the guard, arranged to show us around. By the way, this is . . .'

'I'd better be going,' interjected the young woman, 'I have an appointment.'

She turned abruptly and scurried towards the door, her high heels producing a more feminine version of the click and scrape sound which Peter found quite seductive. Max beamed as the attractive figure approached and, on opening the door for her, he was rewarded with a somewhat mischievous smile. Peter also remained engrossed in the retreating figure. Ben used the few moments to regain his composure, then spoke more soberly as he extended his hand.

'Welcome. I hope that you don't find the horror shift too tedious.'

'I'm used to staying up late,' replied Peter and began to follow as Ben moved towards a nearby corridor. Peter glanced back towards the entrance, hoping perhaps that the young woman might reappear. In so doing her presence was belatedly registered on Ben's conscience.

'Was that girl with you?' he asked.

'No. At least she was here when I arrived and Max showed us around together. She's a student, I believe . . .'

Ben didn't appear interested in any further detail — not that Peter had any to offer — and the subject was changed.

'How long do you plan to work here, Peter?'

'About twelve months if you'll have me. At least I've deferred my course for a year. I need to earn some money.'

'You're most welcome,' continued Ben, 'especially if you don't mind doing some of this night work.'

'As I said . . . it doesn't worry me.'

Ben led the way down to the bunker-like area which contained a vast array of humming and blinking technology. The anxious, bustling, apologetic person whom Peter first encountered upstairs was soon transformed into a likeable, friendly and, in Peter's opinion, extremely intelligent individual. Peter couldn't help remarking upon his early assessment of Ben's abilities.

'How come you are working down here, if you don't mind me saying? You seem a bit too smart for this routine stuff.'

Ben smiled, accepting the compliment graciously as he replied.

'Thanks. It's a long story. I might even bore you with it sometime over the next twelve months.'

However, it would be sooner, much sooner that Peter would learn of the unfortunate circumstances whereby Ben's talent had been consigned to such a mundane institution. Much sooner, indeed, would Peter also become embroiled in a revisitation of those circumstances. His own young analytical brain would be presented with an intriguing challenge which would far transcend the initial drudgery of his new employment.

Ben had worked in the same area for approximately five years, though at different times of the day. He took his turn on the night shift in spite of his relative seniority, partly as it was more tranquil than the day shift and also because it allowed him more free time to pursue other activities. However, this night other activities were put aside as he chatted freely to his new colleague.

Some hours into the night Ben swivelled around to face Peter, turning his back on a monitor which had previously occupied his attention. Peter wore a languid expression which suddenly altered; his eyes focused to the rear of Ben and he contorted his neck slightly to obtain a clearer view. Without even noticing Ben's puzzled response, Peter left his chair and walked, seemingly entranced, towards Ben's monitor. As Peter crouched, a flashing band of numbers was projected across his face.

Ben's puzzled expression momentarily changed to a frown as he turned to see what had captured Peter's attention. Meanwhile Peter spoke. 'Sorry, Ben, I was distracted by your monitor!'

On catching sight of the display, Ben's eyes widened. Then he sprang like a panther, startling his younger colleague.

'That number, I know it!' he gasped.

Peter was promptly displaced by a hip and shoulder movement, causing him to momentarily overbalance. Oblivious to the encroachment, Ben uttered another rasping exclamation. 'The DSP call sign . . . How?'

Now Peter's eyes widened. DSP, or Deep Space Probe, was an expedition which had embarked over six years previously. In fact Peter had only been thirteen years old at the time. The whole mission had been controversial, criticised as too ambitious, if not foolhardy. But its spirit had captivated the imagination of the young and the adventurous, Peter being one such youngster who had followed every phase of the journey. Then, approximately twelve months into the mission, communications were suddenly broken and no trace of the craft ever identified. The critics had their inevitable field day, but apart from that, no one could ever explain why the craft had inexplicably appeared to explode without warning. One could only assume that a major disaster, such as a collision with a meteor or a major malfunction, had befallen the ill-fated crew. No débris was ever identified. Nothing. The popular press speculated about sabotage, black holes, even time warps and other supernatural phenomena, but the scientific community was at a complete loss to explain what had happened.

The designers of the mission were vilified unmercifully, particularly by the media, who indulged in a seemingly endless campaign of pompous hindsight. The loss of the twenty crew members and the huge financial cost of the mission provided their obvious targets.

But people forgot over a period of six years and the whole sordid affair had all but disappeared from even the back pages, apart from occasional reports from clairvoyants who claimed to have received 'messages' from various members of the DSP crew.

Ben had been a high-ranking assistant in the programme and much of the technical design was the result of his painstaking work. Unfortunately, no one escaped the vicious purge which followed the disaster and Ben, like all others associated with the mission, found themselves suddenly suspended, then unemployed. His current position was a far cry from those heady days, but his talents, and indeed those of many of the other scientists, had been recognised by another ambitious individual who had mustered many of them into his fledgling communications business.

Peter eventually plucked up the courage to speak, causing Ben to jump with surprise, Ben's mind clearly absorbed with his flashing numbers which appeared to beg for a response.

'What does it mean?' asked Peter.

'Grab the phone book, Pete,' came the inappropriate reply.

'The phone book! Which phone book?' asked Peter, who had become quite perplexed at the strange turn of events.

Ben managed a faint smile before replying. 'I'm sorry, it's probably some malfunction or . . . a practical joke. I'm amazed I could become so excited after all these years.'

'What's with the phone book?' asked Peter, shrugging his shoulders, 'and did you say something about the DSP?'

'Yes,' replied Ben. Then he paused to let out a long sigh. 'All transmissions began with that call sign, I'm sure of it.'

'So what is it doing in the system here?'

'Well, I presume that its recognition was never cancelled or erased or whatever. You see, a lot of redundant technology was sold off to this company.'

'Was it always the DSP which sent the code?' continued the intrigued Peter.

'Yes. Then a few commands were entered and the signal boosted, especially as the probe travelled further away.'

'So could anyone send a similar signal?'

'Yes, theoretically, that's why I suspect it's a practical joke.'

As Ben's enthusiasm waned, Peter's was kindled. He continued, 'How can we find out? Can we see if there is a message to follow?'

Ben laughed. 'Yeah . . . probably HAPPY APRIL FOOL'S DAY.'

'Except that it's the middle of June,' retorted Peter.

'Let's have the phone book Pete.'

Seeing Peter's renewed puzzlement, Ben continued, 'To obtain the information requires a few instructions that probably only exist in people's memories, or are buried in some completely inaccessible files.'

'So you'll ring . . .?'

'So I'll ring someone who knows, or at least might still remember.'

'Who?' said Peter, now burning with curiosity.

'Joe Sullivan,' sighed Ben as he contemplated phoning the long discredited and retired former director of the DSP mission.

'I should know his number,' mumbled Ben, 'I always mix up the last two digits and I don't wish to wake up the wrong person.'

Although discredited, Joseph Sullivan was not the broken man one might have predicted. Instead he had turned his brilliant mind to, of all things, rose-breeding, and profited to the point whereby he had become an acknowledged expert on the subject, leaving the apparent disgrace of the DSP mission behind him.

The phone rang and rang; rose-breeders were obviously not accustomed to early morning calls. The receiver was eventually lifted and a croak greeted Ben's ear.

'Joe? It's Ben. Ben Andrews!'

A confused dialogue ensued as Ben struggled to identify himself, or at least Joe attempted to elevate his conscious state to the level of comprehension. Ben stated the reason for his untimely call. Silence was his immediate answer.

'I think he's gone back to sleep,' whispered Ben, half turning to Peter.

'No, I haven't,' came a more lucid reply, 'I understand you, Ben. To proceed is a bit complicated. Can I come over?'

'I think it is probably a practical joke, Joe,' replied Ben.

'Who would bother after all these years, and who would remember the call sign?' asked Joe.

'I did,' said Ben. 'Obviously someone else knows that I would have remembered, hence the idea; sour grapes I wonder. We did have our enemies.'

'We sure did, Ben. Anyway, I'll never be able to go back to sleep now without knowing. My curiosity has been aroused. Where exactly are you?'

Ben gave directions and they arranged to meet at the gate to facilitate Joe's passage through security.

Joe replaced the receiver and returned to his somnolent wife, whose desire for slumber took precedence over attempting to comprehend her husband's explanations. Joe then threw on some clothes and set off for the communications centre.

Ben spirited Joe through the communications building to the 'bunker' in the basement. Peter rose as the two entered the room, and was introduced by Ben. Peter recognised Joe, having watched his innumerable television appearances in the past. He noted that this was a more relaxed individual than the one who had borne the strained expression when defending himself against the relentless accusations of his adversaries.

'Pleased to meet you,' said Peter, slightly in awe. 'Ben warned me that this job might be boring and I wind up meeting the director of the Deep Space Probe.'

'Former director,' corrected Joe with a grin.

'This is Peter's first night,' said Ben. 'He's probably going to expect some excitement every night now that this has happened. Apart from that I expect he thinks that I am completely daft.'

The two former colleagues deposited themselves in front of the screen. Peter was relegated to the second row. After a few false starts, and assistance from Ben, Joe managed to find his way around the keyboard. The blinking call sign finally disappeared and the screen went blank.

'Won't be a minute,' murmured Joe. His mind hummed with anticipation. Had some piece of the spacecraft, containing a transmitter, suddenly taken it upon itself to send messages? Or was it a practical joke as Ben had suggested? Such straightforward explanations were to be denied them, however, as the screen suddenly became intensely bright and remained that way. They all stared at the void for what seemed like half an hour before speaking, though in reality it was only about three minutes. Finally Ben said, 'Do you think anything is coming, Joe?'

Joe's face was a map of puzzlement. He turned away from the screen. 'Well, I don't think a practical joker would bother sending us a burst of light or energy.'

'Perhaps it's a recording of the explosion,' said Peter, trying to be helpful.

Many possibilities flicked through Joe's mind. His brow became increasingly furrowed, testifying to the unsatisfactory nature of most of them. Ben broke Joe's concentration with another question. 'Joe?'

'Huh?' came the reply as Joe snapped back to the conversation.

'What exactly was the last transmission from the DSP? I mean, was it like we have just seen, the call sign followed by a white out?'

'No . . . No, in fact Adam, the commander in chief, was transmitting normally, though at a crucial stage of the mission, then everything went completely blank . . . Nothing. It was our astronomers who detected the huge explosion.'

A staccato type of conversation ensued, consisting of odd remarks and grunted replies, interspersed with long periods of silence. The three puzzled members of the group occasionally turned to the screen which steadfastly refused to reveal any further information.

Finally, after about half an hour, the screen went blank and returned to normal transmission. Joe and Ben maintained their perplexed expressions whilst Peter now appeared to become lost in thought. Ben felt Peter's intense concentration.

'OK Pete, what does your young brain make of that?'

'Can we replay it?'

'What! You want to watch thirty minutes of blank screen again? What good will that do?'

'Perhaps we could modify the image or something. There might be something hidden.'

'Hidden?'

'Yes . . . I . . . I thought for a second, just as the screen lit up . . . well I thought I saw an image.'

Ben looked at Joe, who shrugged.

'Can't say that I saw anything,' came Joe's answer to Ben's implied question. 'However, the problem could be that this apparatus may not be able to receive it.'

Ben retrieved the transmission and commenced the replay. The group watched the call sign disappear again, followed by the blank screen. They blinked as the brightness reappeared. Ben paused the recording and spoke.

'I hate to admit it, Pete, but I don't think I saw anything.'

Peter frowned, 'I'm not sure that I did this time,' he said apologetically.

'Slow it down Ben,' suggested Joe.

Back to the start went the recording, an air of disappointment settling over the group once more. However, this time, after concentrating intently, all three reacted with exclamations of hope.

'I think I saw something! . . . Yes . . . definitely . . .'

Back went the recording again.

'Let's take it frame by frame,' said Ben. He replayed the recording yet again, jabbing at the pause sequencer as the vital point approached. After several frames of fuzziness a definite, though blurred, picture appeared. Joe's jaw dropped and he let out an exclamation.

'It's Adam . . . It's a picture of Adam!'

They studied the image intently for a minute. Then Ben

clicked on three more frames similar to the first. Then the brightness took over. Ben returned to the clearest picture and they studied it closely.

Ben and Joe had no difficulty in recognising Adam Coleman, the Deep Space Probe's commander in chief. His image initiated a torrent of memories, many of them painful. Yet the possibility of an explanation for the disappearance of the craft and its crew induced a wave of excitement and anticipation. Ben eventually voiced the thoughts of the group.

'Well! I guess we've somehow picked up his last appearance before disintegration.'

'That would be the obvious explanation . . . I guess,' replied Joe.

Peter shuddered slightly at the thought of witnessing the dreadful destruction, even though it was so long ago in the past. Ben looked at Joe; he could tell that something was puzzling him.

'I'm sorry, Joe. I feel as if I've brought you here on a wild goose chase.'

'No . . . No . . . Don't apologise, Ben, there's nothing like a bit of excitement at my age . . . I guess I should let you two get back to work, that seems to be the end of the transmission. Can you keep a recording and perhaps we could re-examine it at a more respectable hour?'

'Yes, of course,' replied Ben, 'how about you, Pete?'

'Definitely!' said Peter enthusiastically, unable to hide the fact that he was consumed with curiosity.

As Joe departed, Ben and Peter attempted to return to their normal duties, a difficult task given the revelation they had witnessed. It would be some hours before the subject was changed.

'Who did you say that girl was, Peter?' asked Ben, suddenly remembering the individual he had ignored when he first arrived.

'The girl with me at the desk? She said she was a student. Her name's Corinna. Apart from that I don't know anything.'

'Strange,' replied Ben.

'Why? Don't you have students visiting here normally?'

'Yes we do. Some for work experience, others with special interests. But usually during the day, and with one of the senior staff in tow.'

Peter shrugged and continued. 'She was chatting to Max when I arrived. He seemed to think everything was above board. Then she tagged along. We came down here briefly, then we went back upstairs and had a cup of coffee. It wasn't all that long before you appeared.'

Ben stared blankly ahead as the mysterious DSP transmission once again overtook his thoughts. Peter was also silent for a few minutes then piped up again.

'There's one other thing I know about that girl!'

'Huh . . . there is?' replied Ben laconically. 'What's that?'

'Her phone number,' said Peter with a twinkle in his eye.

'Oh I see,' said Ben with a laugh.

'Well . . . she was attractive . . . and had a rather stunning body . . .'

'I get the picture,' said Ben. 'I was in such a hurry I hardly noticed her. Anyway, doesn't a handsome young lad like you already have a girlfriend?'

'Yes sort of,' replied Peter doubtfully, 'but things haven't been going so well lately.'

2

Joe sat on a small dais facing a small band of enthusiastic rose gardeners. His new found interest had lost its appeal in the light of the events of the previous night. His gaze continually wandered upwards to the clear blue sky, scanning back and forth as if he hoped to be suddenly struck by the answer to the riddle.

A rendezvous with his other two witnesses to the extraordinary transmission had been arranged for that afternoon at 4 p.m. Joe's attention eventually came down from the heavens and focused on a portly gentleman who had been expounding on compost, cuttings and insecticides. Joe became vaguely aware of his own name being mentioned along with the fact that he would now speak.

Joe rose from his hard wooden seat, much to the relief of his posterior, and walked robotishly to the centre of the small dais. He spoke in short disjointed sentences, obviously having difficulty concentrating on his subject. Gloria, Joe's wife, wondered why he kept looking up at the sky when all of his life, while speaking in public, he had a habit of dropping his gaze between sentences and when lost for words.

Joe glanced at his watch as he finished his discourse, oblivious to the polite applause which followed.

'4 p.m. seems like light years away,' he murmurred to himself. He frowned. His words seemed to have a strange significance.

His mind swam back many years.

* * *

2020

'But it's light years away!' exclaimed the government minister from behind an intimidatingly large desk.

'I know,' said Joe '. . . Columbus probably said the same to Queen Isabella when she asked him to discover America.'

The politician laughed. 'I don't think your history is too accurate, Joe. It just seems a bit ambitious to go all that way and . . .'

The animated discussion continued with no worthwhile conclusion and in due course Joe left far from satisfied. He wished at that point that all the great explorers and men and women of ambition would reappear to support his case and that of his scientific team.

A deep space probe was hardly a new idea. The multigovernment space agency had been working towards it for twenty years. It seemed that as the possibility of it coming to fruition loomed, those in charge had begun to get cold feet and lose their nerve.

Joe was no blind adventurer; he had meticulously planned every phase of his contribution to the DSP.

All respected Joe's judgement. He had personally overseen the technical aspects of the craft which was to go beyond the solar system. It was the 'human' factor which jeopardised the mission. All previous manned missions within the solar system had been preceded by 'trial runs' with automated technology. To send a craft 'beyond the barrier' and approach the nearest stars would require the control of humans.

Shortage of willing members to crew the DSP was not a problem. But, although those with ultimate responsibility for their fate had developed the jitters, others, including Joseph Sullivan, who had worked long and hard for the climax, harangued, bullied and cajoled their detractors.

The final preparations degenerated into faction fighting, once again over the 'human' factor.

Who should go? How many men, how many women, married or single, how many scientists, how many doctors? Should entertainers be included to relieve boredom? Twenty years of technical preparation seemed trifling compared to these 'human' arguments.

Joe's mind returned to the present. He found himself in the car with Gloria. Normally he drove. This day he relaxed in the passenger seat. Gloria maintained silence; a nagging wife she wasn't. By keeping her mouth closed she found that Joe was much more likely to open his and spill the beans eventually, especially as he could always trust her to be discreet. After ten minutes or so Joe said, 'I suppose you are wondering where I went in the early hours of the morning.'

'A call from a rose bush in need of compost? Or perhaps a visit to an old girl friend,' tittered Gloria.

Joe laughed. With a wife like Gloria, who needs a girlfriend? he thought.

'No. Ben called from the communications centre. They received a transmission from the DSP.'

The normally unruffable Gloria shrieked and pulled the car over to the side of the road, startling the unfortunate motorist behind them. Gloria was oblivious to his cries as he swerved to avoid their vehicle.

'I told you, I told everyone, they would turn up one day, I told them ... I told them!'

Indeed it was true. Gloria had 'told them'. She was a force to be reckoned with if anyone criticised her husband.

Her incisive answers had destroyed many a foe.

'Where are they?' continued Gloria.

'Oh! They're meeting me at 4 p.m.,' replied Joe laconically, his planned meeting with Ben and Peter foremost in his mind. Gloria's puzzled expression triggered a reconsidered reply.

'Oh! I'm sorry, love, you mean the DSP crew.'

Poor Gloria, her ears twitched with desire for information. Joe then recounted the strange event of the night before.

Meanwhile the other two members of the trio had not been idle. Whilst Joe had been expounding on the subject of roses, Ben, after reading a science report on page 5 of a morning newspaper, was rummaging about again for a phone book.

The spreadeagled newspaper lay on the floor. At the bottom of page 5, there was a brief report from a local observatory: *astronomers are puzzled by the appearance of a bright object in the sky for the first time. It appears to have arisen quite suddenly and does not have any of the characteristics of a comet nor other known object,* ... The reporter's own speculations completed the story.

After several frustrating attempts, Ben made contact with a colleague at the observatory.

'Dick? It's Ben Andrews ... We met at a congress in February.'

The voice at the other end acknowledged the occasion and began to confirm events which had occurred at the conference. Ben interrupted, impatient to get to the point of his call.

'It's about a report that I read in today's paper about a bright object that you lot have discovered.'

'Pardon? ...' answered Dick, not surprisingly, as Ben's words had tumbled out in unintelligible haste.

Ben drew breath and repeated the statement. Dick, who

possessed a personality characterised by methodical patience, replied in an irritatingly slow manner to Ben who was clearly desperate for information.

'Ah yes, most interesting, Ben . . . I say, you work in data collection don't you, have you received something unusual?'

Ben did not wish to elaborate on his motives for calling. He answered the question indirectly by saying that it was the newspaper article which prompted the enquiry. Dick continued, prefacing every response with an 'Ah yes' which had the effect of irritating the impatient Ben.

'Ah yes, most fascinating, Ben, the object literally materialised from nowhere . . .'

Dick and Ben both spoke at once wasting more precious seconds.

'Go ahead, sorry, Dick . . .'

Dick recommenced with another 'Ah yes', drawing an almost audible groan from Ben, '. . . but a most extraordinary thing has happened . . .'

A pause followed, Ben bit his tongue to prevent himself from speaking, realising that to do so would produce an even longer pause and another 'Ah yes.'

Dick produced a slight variation. 'Yes well, after it appeared it immediately divided in two. One part is continuing towards us and a second part is going in the reverse direction.'

'Any ideas what it is?' asked Ben hopefully.

'Ah yes, at least not sure on that one. Basically it is an object with some electromagnetic emission travelling very fast. The interesting thing is that the bit which is travelling backwards is like a stream of newly appearing objects which are blue-shifted.'

Dick could offer no further explanations to Ben, who thanked him for his time. Ben slumped into a chair and started to drift into a fitful sleep amidst dreams of exploding spacecrafts and strange messages.

Meanwhile Peter passed the day visiting libraries and technical bookshops. The events of the previous night had tantalised his young mind, and he returned home with an armful of reading material, ranging from orbital mechanics to relativity theories. It would be his mind that, eventually, would all but solve the riddle.

3

2024

As 2024 dawned, so did the planned launch of the first manned deep space probe. The new century had brought a wave of optimism and euphoria which had been exploited by those with an interest in space exploration. A major factor also had been the absence of any major conflicts around the world for over ten years, which meant that finance, formerly directed to useless weapons and their inevitable destruction of life and property, was now channelled into the major space programmes. Cooperation between nations, which eliminated costly duplication, had also garnished space projects.

Joseph Sullivan, though meticulous in nature, was inspired by the interstellar mission and had risen to become the director of the whole programme. With the support of similarly inspired colleagues, he pressed forward towards the launch date. An approach to the nearest stars had not been ruled out, though it would depend on the endurance of the crew and their supplies. Such an effort would require a round trip time around twenty years, but the final decision would rest with the crew itself. This aspect of the mission was a strict secret, the more modest goal of flying 'as far as one could', then coming back, being the publicised target.

It was the indefinite goal which provided the detractors with their major ammunition. 'People are never happy in this field unless you go somewhere specific and bring back a lump of useless rock!' exclaimed Joe to a colleague during one of the many debates on mission objectives. Fortunately he had the support of the astronomers who translated their desire to examine space from outside the constraints of the solar system into a cause worth fighting for.

Agreement was eventually reached on the objectives. However the final stages then got bogged down in minutiae, not the least of which were arguments over the crew. Joe demanded a large part of this decision and for the most part got his way.

In spite of the failings of human nature, one could only be impressed to the point of wonderment at man's ability to create the complex and magnificent craft that was to explore the unknown. Whilst many great minds and individual efforts had produced the components, one great mind had brought it all together; that of Joseph Sullivan.

As Joe stepped from the Earth shuttle aboard the finished product of his efforts, one could see a man, modest by nature, yet in the prime of his life and unable to conceal the air of an individual flushed with pride and satisfaction. Yet he had an apprehension about what he had created and its ultimate fate and the fate of those who would ride with it. Would the prophets of doom have the last say?

Joe dismissed such thoughts from his mind with the adage: 'Nothing attempted nothing gained.' He then allowed himself to wallow in the magnificence that surrounded him.

Much of the technology on the DSP was untried, in the sense that unlike a new ship which can be sailed around a harbour in order to try it out, this craft would be proven on its maiden voyage. This factor applied particularly to the mainly nuclear-powered engines which were designed to produce velocities which had never been achieved before and, along with this, the consequent control and stability of the craft.

Such apprehensions also existed for the crew, who were to be flung into the unknown for an indeterminable period of time, possibly for ever. Many hopeful individuals had 'practised' enforced hibernation, and the same had been subjected to much scientific and psychological evaluation. Joe, however, discounted much of this practice as a waste of time as such 'rehearsals' were bespoiled by the fact that the hibernators could forestall their situation if it was really necessary. Instead Joe sought out individuals who had survived real life situations, particularly those who had been in a predicament where there had been no light at the end of the tunnel. Even former hostages and kidnap victims suddenly found themselves being contacted by Joe and his staff; not necessarily to join the DSP crew, but because Joe found their thoughts invaluable in the preparation of those who eventually did.

When one thinks of a 'hand picked crew' one thinks of the best in the field. Whilst some were, the majority of Joe's selections were all-rounders. 'It's no good having a genius on board if he goes to pieces in a crisis,' argued Joe repeatedly. So in the exhaustive interviews, Joe would probe for a crisis in the applicant's life; in fact to have had one became a positive advantage. Joe wanted people who had tasted apprehension, fear and disappointment and conquered them.

Joe would dearly have loved to explore the whole craft, but that would have taken weeks. Instead he made straight for the command centre, which in due course would also be called the 'flight deck' by some, or the 'bridge' by others, depending upon their background. The command centre was duplicated for safety reasons. Large screens surrounded the consoles. Apart from projecting important data the screens could also display panoramas of wide open spaces in order to minimise the feeling of claustrophobia for the occupants. The craft would be run essentially on nuclear power with some solar initially, and conventional fuel as a standby.

Various officials accompanied Joe on the tour, plus five key members of the crew. There would be no official democracy on this craft; every individual had a position and had sworn to respect it. Experienced space personnel, however, had learnt that, once away from Earth, individuals became equal, and even if injustice occurred, it was more expedient to accept it than waste time on some sort of artificial judiciary.

After much debate about titles, the commander in chief was simply referred to as 'Captain', a title which would be used more in mock than true respect. Inevitably a group of people, like a family or sporting team or a military unit, would develop their own titles and nicknames. Equality in numbers of each sex was not deliberately sought, but inevitably it occurred by natural selection, proving that men and women are definitely of equal ability.

The navy provided the Captain, Adam Coleman. He was one of the few career military persons on board, though many had performed some sort of part-time military service. Adam was one of Joe's all-rounders, apart from his scientific interests. He was tall, extremely fit and possessed an unshakeable sense of fair play. He had also once survived a shipwreck, thus fulfilling Joe's selection criterion of having overcome a crisis.

Accompanying Adam were his co-commanders: Alex Alexeyeff, essentially a scientist, but also trained in the technical side of the craft, as were the crew in general. Maria Fontana came to the mission by way of her mathematical abilities and flying skills. She was also an above average gymnast, having competed at an Olympic meeting as a teenager. Yvonne Deschamps shared Maria's sporting background only in the field of sailing, an attribute that would draw many quips as to how she would pursue her hobby in space. Her main contribution to the mission, however, would be as a physicist. The fifth member of the group was Jack Donaldson. Jack would lead a team of technicians who would keep the craft in working order. Between them they possessed by far the greatest array of all-round skills amongst the personnel on board. In spite of all the sophisticated equipment, Joe wanted natural brains overseeing the operations.

It was assumed that the physical fitness of the crew, combined with a vegetarian diet, would minimise illness. However, two doctors and two nurses would be on board, though they would spend most of their time assisting in other areas. Botanists and caterers completed the crew, though they also possessed all-round attributes. A total of twenty personnel were to be the final complement on board the DSP.

Joe and his group completed their tour and returned to Earth. After inevitable last minute hitches, time seemed to evaporate and the launch date loomed.

4

The final crew of the DSP assembled. They were addressed by various speakers, including leaders of nations, scientists and special interest groups. Joe Sullivan was eventually given his turn. He knew every member of the crew personally; two in particular were closer than anyone realised. Their imminent departure produced a wrenching feeling, but he composed himself and rationalised his feelings along the lines that if he were feeling emotional about the impending separation, then so must the families and friends of the crew as a whole.

The crew had trained and worked together for many months. A large amount of time was spent on familiarisation and much on exchange of ideas and skills. Euphoria gripped the crew as the launch date approached. One common thread in their personalities, further enhanced when in a group, was optimism. Psychological preparation had concentrated on what could become the two biggest evils, pessimism and petty jealousy. Fears of these potential curses were to prove unnecessary, however.

The launch itself, if anything, was an anticlimax; no spectacular lift off as with craft leaving Earth, just a gentle 'drift off' from the Earth's orbit. Great thrust and speed were to come later.

Six hours into the mission Adam and his co-commanders

sat in the command centre. This and the normal working areas of the craft rotated to provide artificial gravity for most of the day to day activities of the crew. The group chatted amiably, having completed their initial duties. In due course a silence descended. Alex broke it. 'We have a problem my friends, after six hours we have run out of conversation.'

'We could play Scrabble,' remarked Maria innocently, remembering a joint decision by the crew before departure not to bring it in any form.

'It would have to be a long game,' laughed Adam.

'How about throwing a malfunction, Adam?' said Yvonne. 'Just to put everyone on their toes.'

'Deliberate' malfunctions were part of the design of the mission. Their purpose was to test the skills of the crew from time to time.

'Why not?' said Adam with a grin, 'Maria . . . throw a spanner in the works.'

The DSP operated on a twenty-four hour 'day'. Initially there was regular two way communication with Earth, but as the turn around time for responses increased, straight transmissions replaced them. As this happened the crew became more of a closed community. Fear of interpersonal problems between crew members proved unfounded. In fact the reverse was true. Everyone would dearly have loved a bit of gossip or a 'crisis' to natter about.

'I used to criticise sensationalism in the press,' remarked Adam. 'Now I miss it because I can't tut tut about it.'

News from Earth proved no compensation. Fires, floods, and famines, although recognised as disasters on Earth, seemed to have little relevance aboard a spacecraft. Likewise politics became totally irrelevant. The lack of common laws and rules was definitely the most positive aspect of life on board. One didn't miss the hassles of traffic, the danger of dark alleys, nor censorship, nor bigotry.

The crew evolved its own unique lifestyle. Apart from conventional type exercise and activity, groups would travel to the weightless areas in the main shafts which abutted the fore and aft engine complexes. Tending the huge gardens proved a therapeutic and relaxing activity enjoyed by all. Athough generally bound by a rigid self-discipline in their normal duties, the crew were renowned for their 'antics' especially in the weightless areas, where variations of popular sports were enacted with hilarious results. One uninhibited group indulged in a memorable game of 'frisbee', memorable because the uninhibited aspect of the recreation included removing their clothes which hung like barrage balloons to impede the path of the perpetually motioned missile. Someone had activated a 'spy camera' and the match was replayed on numerous occasions much to the embarassment of the participants. It remained the high point of the voyage for many months.

There was much rotation amongst the crew and special interest meetings. Inevitably the forthcoming superacceleration became a major topic of discussion. Richard Johnson (commonly known as Bud) was second in command to Jack Donaldson, the chief technician. He and a group of others picked Yvonne's brains:

'Do you think that we will approach the speed of light?' questioned Bud.

Yvonne shrugged and replied. 'Well, it's theoretically possible; as long as we apply more thrust, we increase our speed.'

'Yes, but don't we become incredibly heavy as we travel faster?' chimed in Henny, one of the caterers.

Bernard, one of the techs, laughed. 'Trust a cook to worry about our weight. You'll just have to put us on a diet, Henny!'

Yvonne continued after the laughter had died down.

'Our mass as distinct from our weight increases, it's true, but only gradually at first. It is only near the speed of light that it really increases dramatically and approaches infinity.'

'How near?' asked Henny.

'Well, at half the speed of light, it is only 1.15 times our original mass and at three quarters light speed it is one and a half times.'

'So when do we get really heavy?' continued Henny, eager to get to the end point of the discussion.

'Heaviness is another thing,' replied Yvonne, wishing once again to avoid confusion between weight and mass. 'At nine tenths light speed, mass is 3.33 times normal, and at 0.99 light speed it is seven times normal.'

A pause followed whilst the group digested Yvonne's facts and figures. Bud took over the explanations. 'Our mass is really irrelevant anyway, if we are all accelerating at the same rate.'

'Exactly,' said Yvonne, 'it is only when one is accelerating in a gravitational field that we feel any force or weight, like when we feel the G forces as we accelerate away from Earth.'

'How close do you think we will go?' asked Bud.

'That's still to be determined,' said Yvonne. 'We'll be analysing data as we go, but I know that we have been briefed to approach light speed if possible.'

Henny looked slightly indignant. 'It makes you feel a bit like a guinea pig, doesn't it!'

Bud laughed. 'Relax Henny, think of how much more quickly we will complete the journey.'

'I'd like to complete it in one piece,' said Henny, a slight smirk creeping onto her face to show that she didn't take the discussion too seriously. 'I think I've been locked up with a bunch of mad scientists!'

'Don't worry Henny,' said Yvonne, 'trust us . . . at these

high speeds you'll be back in time to shake hands with yourself as you are leaving.'

The casualness of the earlier part of the journey departed along with the solar system which the DSP eventually left behind. The crew prepared for acceleration to speeds never dreamed of before. Much was to be done. Even though most of the manoeuvre would be computer-guided, the crew would supervise closely. Joe Sullivan had placed great faith in his 'humans' to keep an eye on the machines. The thrust would be applied in stages with pauses for evaluation.

As an amalgam of people and machine coalesced, Adam and Alex surveyed a screen full of data.

'I suppose we should be careful of the "beach" syndrome,' muttered Adam.

'The "beach" syndrome?' replied a puzzled Alex.

'Yes. Remember when you were young, the sun was shining and you were heading for the beach with your surfboard in the rear of your car,' continued Adam wearing a rather idyllic expression.

'One didn't surf where I came from,' said Alex in a deflated manner.

Adam continued, 'The temptation was to drive faster and faster in order to arrive as soon as possible.'

'Now I understand,' said Alex. 'Were you really a surfer though?'

'Wouldn't know one end of a wave from another,' laughed Adam, 'but it's a good analogy, don't you think?'

'Not bad. At least I can't think of a better one,' said Alex as he turned his attention back to his duties.

'To be honest, Adam, I don't expect any problems with the acceleration.'

'In that case I'll load the surfboard.'

As the two chuckled, Anna Bryant had crept into the command centre. Anna was one of the two doctors on board, though she also assisted Carl Schmidt and Tony

Borsari, the two botanists.

'What amuses you two? Is this the euphoria prior to our disintegration?' she asked with a smirk creeping across her face.

'Anna believes that as we approach light speed, gravitational forces will cause us to be attracted to each other,' said Alex with a twinkle in his eye.

'And distintegrate?' said Adam with a note of seriousness.

'Actually Carl and Tony are worried about the effect on their plants,' said Anna.

'Don't worry, Anna, tell the guys that if their oranges start showing the slightest bit of affection for each other, I'll take my foot off the gas,' said Adam.

'But what if we can't control the power?' said Anna somewhat prophetically.

The two men were momentarily silent. Anna had in a few words summed up the fragility of their existence. However, she suddenly realised that she was breaking a cardinal rule: voicing doubt and pessimism. She quickly corrected herself.

'I'm sorry, guys . . . just playing devil's advocate.'

Adam spoke authoritatively: 'No, don't apologise Anna, you know that I welcome ideas that make us think, it helps us to anticipate.'

Anna excused herself, leaving Adam and Alex to their deliberations. She visited Maria and recounted her recent conversation with Maria's co-commanders. Maria, unable to resist a mathematical challenge, seized on Anna's ideas.

'You realise that you have posed one of the major questions that we have been chartered to answer,' said Maria.

'You mean, see what happens to a tin full of humans travelling at the speed of light or thereabouts?'

'You think we are guinea pigs, Anna?'

'No of course not. At least I realise that we are sort of. I mean one has to be, if we are to explore the unknown.'

'One can explore the unknown without being foolish, Anna, and we have no intentions of doing anything blatantly dangerous.'

Anna was silent, so Maria continued, 'Don't worry, Anna, everyone on board has become a bit jittery. I am having similar conversations with many people.'

Anna raised a smile and spoke. 'Who makes the key decisions if the going gets rough?'

'Adam . . . and only Adam. He has total command, otherwise we would have different scientists all suggesting conflicting courses of action.'

Others approached the same subject in a more light-hearted manner. Henny Jacobs and her two assistant caterers, Gerda and Paul, pronounced their theories.

'I reckon that we will reach the speed of light,' pontificated Paul, folding his arms as if to lend weight to the validity of his pronouncement.

'Yeah, sure . . . then we will be able to see right through each other,' remarked Gerda.

'Henny, if that's the case I'll be able to see your knickers,' said Paul cheekily.

'You won't see mine,' said Gerda with a wicked look, as she flounced out of the room with a plate of hors d'oeuvres. She turned her head as she left and smirked at her puzzled colleagues. 'I don't wear any.'

'Really,' said Henny, pretending to be shocked.

'I'm sure it will be interesting, though,' continued Paul, obviously enjoying the speculation. 'Your meals might glow in the dark, Henny!'

'I suspect that nothing will happen at all,' said Henny more soberly, deflating Paul's fantasies somewhat.

'Oh Henny, how dull you are, where's your imagination?'

Henny just smiled and handed Paul a platter of artistically arranged vegetables and fruit.

Paul smiled. 'Silly me. Fancy accusing you of having no imagination, Henny.'

'You let those scientists worry about our speed, Paul. If they can produce food like this for us to work with in the middle of a vacuum, I've no doubt that they know what they are doing.'

Meanwhile Anna and Maria completed their conversation with a different conclusion.

'Such blind faith,' said Anna.

'You mean in Adam?' replied Maria.

'No,' said Anna, '. . . in science.'

5

David Simpson was Anna's medical partner on the voyage. The two had also come to form a more intimate relationship along with the professional one. They lay sprawled across the bed, staring at the ceiling.

'You know, I've been worried about this light speed business,' said Anna languidly, giving the impression that she was anything but worried.

'So I gather,' replied David, 'you've been obsessed with it.'

'Just trying to sort things out in my own mind. Now I'm quite fascinated; in fact I'm interested to see if we actually pass it.'

'We can't pass it, Anna, it's an ultimate figure!'

Anna possessed no respect for scientific machinations. She often had great delight in pointing to famous scientists throughout history who had enunciated the absolute, only to have their hallowed beliefs disproven at a later date. David had known Anna well enough and long enough to recognise her mood. It was one in which she was about to challenge the established order.

'I read once, that everyone made a big fuss about the sound barrier. Well, breaking the light barrier is just the next step.'

'I think the light barrier, as you call it, is a little different,' declared David.

'What's the speed of sound?' demanded Anna.

'I feel as if I'm about to provide the evidence that will ultimately convict me,' said David with a laugh. Anna stared at David with a devilish smile, sitting up as she did so.

'It's about 500 to 600 miles per hour,' said David reluctantly, 'and to answer your next question, the speed of light is 186,000 miles per second.'

'I already know that. It's the speed of sound that I always seem to have trouble remembering. Anyway, the point is that they are both finite numbers.'

'So?'

'So the only ultimate number is infinity. If it's possible to pass 500, then it's possible to pass 186,000.'

Anna folded her arms in obvious satisfaction, even though she knew that her pronouncements probably had no scientific merit. David realised that the argument was flawed, but his scientific knowledge was inadequate to point out the error.

Without prolonging the discussion the two fell asleep, as if exhausted by all the brain work. Anna slept with the smug satisfaction of an individual who has won a contest by the use of dirty tricks. David, on the other hand, felt like an individual who had held a winning hand at cards, but somehow had lost the game.

Most general assemblies of the crew were for social reasons. However, everyone knew that the next one would herald a new dimension in the journey. Adam addressed the group with a little more formality than usual. Nevertheless he still managed to inspire a relaxed type of confidence in his crew. His manner provided the invisible glue which held morale together. He first presented some routine data and results of analyses so far. He was aware that his crew understood the overall principles of relativity and the possibilities as their speed increased. Indeed most of the crew had discussed little else in recent weeks.

'The critical time will occur in a few days,' said Adam bluntly, his eyes darting around to gauge the reaction.

He waited for his audience to digest the statement. However there was little reaction, certainly no murmuring, nudging nor other signs of overt apprehension.

Eventually Anna said, 'Don't worry Adam, we've all reached the stage where we are dying to see what happens!'

Exclamations of enthusiasm and concurrence followed Anna's pronouncement. Adam appeared a little less starchy. He continued, 'Very well, we'll be applying thrust in stages as usual, so I'll hit the brakes if anything odd happens. I want the non-technical crew members paired with Jack's team, firstly to assist, as you are used to doing when necessary, and secondly so that the techs can keep you informed as to what is happening at all stages. As you are aware, we are not in a gravitational field, so we don't expect anything terribly unusual.'

Adam then deferred to Jack, who said, 'There will be two sets of co-commanders then, Adam and Maria, and Alex and Yvonne. Actually, David will join the first group and Anna the second, the rest of you will be paired as follows: Carl with me, Tony with Bud, Loretta with Helen, Kate with Carmel, Henny with Stephanie, Gerda with Alan, and Paul with Bernard.'

'Thanks Jack,' said Adam, 'I'd say any questions, but as we probably don't have the answers, I won't bother.'

With that the crew dispersed.

Fuelled by weeks of speculation and anticipation the crew of the DSP manned their stations. David and Anna, although officially assigned to the command areas, adopted a more floating role which included preparing the virtually unused clinical area of the craft.

Yvonne stared intently at her feet. Alex had noticed the interest in her extremeties and remarked, 'Counting your toes in case some fall off?'

'No,' she replied immediately, 'I was trying to imagine myself in high heels again.'

'Yes. We do tend to be practical rather than fashionable. Don't worry, Yvonne, we might come across a nice interstellar shopping mall.'

Yvonne gave a deep sigh with an air of resignation. 'I'll be too old to then . . .'

Alex interrupted her with a laugh. 'Poor old Grandma, over the hill already. Don't worry, old girl, all this high speed travel will make you younger.'

Yvonne started to smile but she suddenly shot a glance at Alex. From the expression on her face, it was obvious that it had nothing to do with their frivolous conversation, but an almost imperceptable sudden movement which Yvonne's astute nature recognised as being abnormal. She stood bolt upright.

'Our acceleration rate has changed,' she stated.

'What do you mean?' asked Alex, looking mystified.

'I don't know. Something has happened.'

They both immediately focused on the display monitors. They had become alive. Yvonne's eyes fixed on their speed. It was racing at an incomprehensible rate, something it certainly should not be doing.

Alex joined Yvonne and stared at the incomprehensible display. For some reason he then turned and looked behind, somehow sensing that an answer to the numerous questions, which suddenly racked his brain, might appear. He gasped at what met his eyes.

'Yvonne! Look behind!'

'What the . . .!'

Yvonne shot a glance behind her. She and Alex both stared towards the corridor. It appeared to bend, initially, then go dull as the colours of the fittings appeared to separate like a picture on a 3-D comic page. Yvonne quickly spun back the other way, which corresponded to the direction in which they were travelling. In this direction everything appeared clear, though somewhat brighter, she thought.

Meanwhile, Jack stared at a myriad of malfunctions. He desperately tried to focus his thoughts towards some sort of meaningful response and, at the same time, remain calm. Adam's image suddenly appeared on a screen before him. Adam wore an expression of concern that looked quite alarming. He was about to speak to Jack when he turned in response to a stifled gasp from Maria.

'Adam, look out!'

As Adam spun, he saw a wall of blackness racing towards them from the rear, engulfing everything in its path, and before he could even utter an exclamation, Maria had vanished.

Communications between the DSP and Earth now took months in each direction. From recent transmissions, however, Joe Sullivan knew that the craft would soon be entering the crucial stage of acceleration, and he and his staff watched around the clock in anticipation. They could do nothing but watch, helpless, in that they no longer had any influence; everything was in Adam's hands. Of course what they were about to witness had already happened months ago by the time the details reached Earth. Joe and his colleagues watched entranced, their minds choked with anticipation.

'I guess this is the moment we've been waiting for,' said Joe ruefully. By nature Joe was a methodical character. He believed in careful planning which aimed at eliminating, or at least minimising risk. He had long argued for a 'maximum' safe speed for the DSP. He regarded the flirtation near light speed as an unnecessary experimentation. Reluctantly he had bowed to pressure from his advisers.

Now it was happening, at least for the spectators on Earth; for the DSP it was all over. Joe and his group watched the speed increase incrementally. Joe pictured the equally methodical Adam pausing whilst he evaluated the response of the craft. Adam would be in the command centre, of course. It didn't seem all that long ago that Joe had stood there himself with Adam and the other senior members of the crew. Joe prayed that Adam would make the right decisions and back off if anything unusual happened. He suddenly became aware of exclamations of wonderment around him.

'Wow . . . it's happening!'

'Can you believe it?'

'How much closer?'

Streams of data surged into computers. The disciples of relativity gobbled it up like starved dogs.

Then it happened. With the help of the astronomers they determined that it took the form of a huge flash. Closer analysis demonstrated that it was a giant nuclear explosion, easily one hundred kilometres in diameter. With the amount of nuclear fuel on board the DSP, such a catastrophe was quite feasible.

The holocaust gradually faded, though 'hot spots' continued to show for some hours, but no other transmission. The DSP had been equipped with black box type transmitters, but it was assumed that these would have been consumed in the explosion.

Joe's only words were 'Oh no!'

Others cried. Most were bewildered, and inevitably, when the news got out, the seeds of a witch hunt germinated in the minds of adversaries. Certain politicians and newspaper editors had given little support to the DSP project, though had managed to poise themselvses cunningly to take advantage of it, if the time came. They specialised in making ambiguous statements which could be interpreted as being either for or against. Their eventual position would be dictated by the success or failure of the mission. That point being determined, they now loaded their guns. The initial tone was one of 'we told you so' but more ruthless individuals cashed in on the publicity by prolonging it in order to demand retribution. One particular newspaper editor, named Jenkins, almost persuaded equally hysterical politicians to press criminal charges against Joe Sullivan and his colleagues. Although opposed to the light speed idea, Joe defended it for the sake of his colleagues. In fact he had convinced himself that it could be made safe by using a careful approach.

'What went wrong?' he repeatedly asked himself.

Many enquiries were held, but with all the publicity and official interrogation there was little time to reflect. Joe and his team were suspended and eventually dismissed. In fact the whole agency had been built around the DSP project and it all but disintegrated, along with the craft itself.

Personal details of the crew had always been kept confidential; now Joe fought to keep them that way. Fortunately he had the considerable support of the families of the crew members. The more senior members of the crew were most vulnerable because aspects of their careers had attracted publicity in the past. Maria's Olympic appearance provided the media with photographs and film which was replayed endlessly.

A stony wall of silence confronted those who enquired about the junior members of the crew. Even before departure, personal details of crew members had been kept secret to prevent unwarranted publicity. Concealing the names, however, was impossible, and most newspapers and television news programs promulgated a list:

Adam Coleman, commander in chief
Alex Alexeyeff, co-commander

Maria Fontana, co-commander
Yvonne Deschamps, co-commander
Jack Donaldson, chief technician
Richard Johnson, senior technician
Helen Fournier, technician
Carmel O'Leary, technician
Alan Gilchrist, technician
Bernard Bichet, technician
Stephanie Griffin, technician
Carl Schmidt, botanist
Antonio Borsari, botanist
David Simpson, doctor
Anna Bryant, doctor
Loretta Spillare, nurse
Katherine Canning, nurse
Henny Jacobs, caterer
Gerda Sternberg, caterer
Paul Wilson, caterer.

The media compensated for their lack of personal information by fabricating as much as they could around snippets of gossip. There were those, of course, who came forward claiming to have known various crew members personally.

The news finally began to subside after many months. Gloria provided a lifeline to sanity for her husband; she also extended her hospitality to Joe's demoralised friends and their families. In the early days after the disaster, Gloria thought that she would restore spirits with a dinner party at which she went to considerable effort to prepare a sumptuous meal, theorising that nourishment for the body would also feed the mind. Although gratefully acknowledged by the forlorn scientists, their appetites were so suppressed that little was eaten. This had the effect of magnifying their guilt and humiliation. However, another attempt was to be made, this time at the instigation of

Gloria and Joe's two daughters, Karen and Millie. Millie was the younger of the two, being thirteen years old. She had spent a considerable portion of her childhood at home with recurrent respiratory complaints. Along with this medical problem she had suffered a chronically poor appetite which also partially explained her wispy and delicate appearance. In order to nourish the waif, her mother had devised simple and tasty titbit style meals. Now Millie reminded Gloria of them as she prepared another onslaught on the scientists' absent appetites.

Karen Sullivan was nineteen and, although never afflicted by het younger sister's childhood ailments, had a similar slender build. The gathering of the demoralised took place on a warm summer evening, which proved a good start in the quest to elevate the spirits. However the group still bore the air of one nursing fractured dreams and purpose. Karen and Millie fluttered about the members of the group like delicate butterflies distributing enchanted nectar and breaking an evil spell. The mood lightened and the bite-sized morsels resurrected dormant appetites and spirits. Ben Andrews attended the gathering. Like the others he had been despondent, though not quite to the same degree; his youth at least offering some hope of re-employment, unlike the prospects of some of his older colleagues. He sat in a low armchair as Karen approached for the first time.

Karen possessed an elegant beauty, he thought; not the voluptuous type, more the ethereal balletic type. Karen stopped directly in front of Ben and leant forward with her platter of irresistables. A beautiful enchanting smile appeared on her face and as she leant forward, the neckline of her light summer frock fell away from her chest. Ben's line of vision came into direct contact with a pair of perfectly shaped unfettered breasts, causing him to audibly gulp, blush and raise his eyes to the equally beautiful smile.

'Th .. Thank you . . .' he stuttered, taking a canapé, then dropping it in his lap. Karen placed her platter on a nearby table, then squatted beside Ben. At the same time she produced a serviette from nowhere, like a conjurer, and to Ben's further embarrassment proceeded to wipe his trousers clean. Like many young scientific enthusiasts, Ben's devotion to his profession determined that experience in relationships with girls had been limited. Later in the evening, when Karen's catering duties subsided, he sought her out and took the first steps along the path of what would ultimately become a permanent relationship.

However the true 'fairy princess' of the evening was undoubtedly Millie. Her determination to make the evening a success had been engraved all over her face. The scientists seemed to have been jolted back to their senses by this unlikely crusader; some even felt slightly ashamed at their previous behaviour and the low morale that it had produced. In any case the evening marked a real turning point. The scientists who possessed such outstanding abilities were to find that not everyone held them in low esteem, and all were to be eventually gainfully employed once more.

And so the years passed and the DSP was all but forgotten. Now the mysterious signal had rekindled the thoughts of Joe, Ben and Peter. They all arrived at their 4 p.m. rendezvous, the lack of sleep showing in their sunken faces, but not in their eyes, which projected, antenna-like, from their sockets.

'I've been staring at the sky all day long,' quipped Joe.

'I have some news,' said Ben, and he produced the newspaper clipping and recounted his conversation with the astronomer.

Peter then put in his bit. 'That's interesting,' he said slowly and then became lost in thought. Joe and Ben looked at him for a moment. Then realising that nothing else was forthcoming, Ben continued, 'Joe . . . when the explosion occurred, there definitely was no débris identified?'

'None . . . I know not all details of the events were released, but I assure you that nothing tangible survived. What are you suggesting, Ben?'

'Well . . . suppose most of it was flung away from us . . . the craft was travelling near the speed of light, hence it's probably not surprising that nothing came towards us.'

Joe thought for a minute. Somehow he seemed more able to discuss the DSP explosion, years later, than he had been able at the time or shortly after. He eventually answered.

'I've often thought along the same lines. Do you think a chunk has somehow done a circuit, like a comet, and is on its way back to us?'

'I know it won't bring the crew back,' continued Ben, 'but it would be great to get some answers. Will you join us on our shift tonight, Joe?'

'I'd be glad to. Do you think anyone knows anything yet?'

'I doubt it. The day shift will naturally record all routine data, but the DSP's call sign wouldn't be recognised amongst everything else and it won't be analysed for a week or more.'

Apart from small talk, the meeting provided nothing else of concrete value and the three decided that sleep was the next priority, especially as they would be burning the midnight oil.

'I'm home!' called Joe as he opened his front door. Gloria rushed to him.

'Any news?' she asked hopefully.

'Nothing in particular. I'm joining Ben and Peter on their night shift again, though.'

'What do you think it is?'

'Well, the best explanation we can come up with, and even then we don't have any real evidence, is that some piece of the craft with a black box transmitter has somehow wound up heading in our direction.'

Gloria looked pleased.

'Wouldn't it be wonderful to have some answers . . . even after all this time . . . just to know what happened.'

Suddenly the front door was assaulted with a loud rapping sound. Joe and Gloria looked at each other.

'Karen!' they exclaimed in unison as they recognised her trademark. Gloria hastened to the door and swung it open to reveal Karen's beaming face.

'Hi! Is Ben here? He left a note saying he was meeting Dad.'

Joe appeared at that point and both parents received an affectionate kiss from their daughter.

'Everything OK?' she stated, her senses bristling.

'Yes, of course honey,' replied Joe. 'Don't worry, Ben's on his way home, we ... er . . . had something to discuss.'

'Sounds serious, Dad. Your roses all sick or something?' Karen wore a mischievous expression as she probed for information.

'Can we tell her, Joe?' asked Gloria.

'Of course,' said Joe, feeling that now he didn't have much choice. 'It's about a DSP signal Ben received last night.'

Karen clasped her hands to her face whilst letting out a shriek.

'The DSP! You're not serious . . . they're coming back . . . Oh!'

Joe smiled at his daughter's fairy tale outlook on life. 'It's not that good, I'm afraid, my dear, but it's possible a transmitter from the craft has turned up and it's heading towards us. It may give us some answers.'

Karen, although deflated, still managed an enthusiastic tone.

'Yeah. Well. That's what I meant, I guess!'

Later that night, Joe, Ben and Peter reassembled. Ben

and Peter put in an hour of frenzied activity, achieving what would normally be spread over about four hours. No new data had appeared with the DSP call sign, so they retrieved the recording from the night before. But no new information could be gleaned.

'Basically a bright spot travelling at incredible speed,' summarised Ben, after they had discussed the astronomical findings again.

An air of disappointment befell them. They had been cheated, their appetites whetted and then the meal cruelly snatched away. Just as despondency reached its zenith, Ben's screen responded to their mental pleas by reproducing the DSP call sign. Ben gave a whoop and seized upon the terminal; then, realising that he needed Joe's assistance, he vacated the seat and allowed him to take over.

But there were to be no images this time, just a sequence of unintelligible transmissions. No amount of modification to the signal produced any further information.

'I believe that our problem lies in the equipment,' stated Joe bluntly.

6

2025

Jack stared at the image of Adam on the intercom and watched as a look of terror swept the captain's face.

'Adam! Adam!' he shouted. 'What is it?'

But Adam didn't seem to hear. Jack turned to his assistants and was immediately hit by a wall of blackness. Meanwhile, Maria stared at Adam. The person whom she regarded as steady as the rock of Gibraltar wore an expression of fear such as she had never encountered. She ran forward to him. He screeched as she touched him. It appeared that he couldn't see her coming.

'Who is it? I can't see!' he screamed.

Maria was suddenly aware of blackness on either side of her. She turned slightly and faced into total darkness, yet when she turned forward all was clear. She quickly came to terms with the phenomenon; even though she had no explanation for it, analysis would have to wait. She grasped Adam firmly and swung him so that she was now in front of him. She felt a shiver as she was engulfed in total darkness.

No wonder Adam had looked terrified, she thought. She spoke with a trembling voice. 'It's all right, Adam, you should be able to see and hear me now. Don't bother to answer, I can't see or hear you. Now we are going to turn again so that you can speak to me, don't let go!'

They rotated 180 degrees. Maria was thankful to be able to see again and surveyed Adam's perplexed expression. He was momentarily lost for words.

'Maria . . . Maria . . . my God . . .' he uttered.

Maria swung him again. She tried to stifle her own fear in order to sound reassuring; facing total darkness didn't help.

'I was the lucky one, Adam, I was facing forward when it struck . . .'

Maria was interrupted as she felt herself pulled around by Adam; he had now grasped the situation.

'OK, OK, I get it. We can see to the front, but not to the rear. How do we . . . I mean what has happened?'

Another rotation brought an answer.

'Adam, we must be outrunning light because . . . because light from behind us can't catch us, so everything is black . . . Whereas light from in front hits us, if anything, faster and brighter. Turn round now and answer me. And can you relax your grip a bit? You're cutting off my circulation!'

'Sorry,' said Adam coming back into Maria's view. 'It's weird talking to a pitch black wall. Thank God I can feel you.'

Adam paused, forgetting that no reply would be forthcoming. Maria reappeared in front of him. 'What do you remember happening when the darkness arrived?'

Adam replied after turning; they now had the manoeuvre down to a fine art.

'I was about to pause acceleration when something propelled us forward at an incredible rate. It all happened so quickly. Next thing I knew this wall of black was heading straight at us!'

'Yes. I saw it coming, but then I turned to tell you . . .

Mama mia! . . . You should have seen the look on your face!'

'I don't wonder,' replied Adam, 'heaven knows what effect all this has had on the rest of the crew.'

'Adam, let's stand side by side and see what we can make of all this . . . say for five minutes . . . then we'll resume our conversation.'

They linked arms and faced forwards. When they peered sidewards the very tips of their extremities projected out of a black wall. Maria shuddered at the macabre picture, and busied herself with the displays before her. A mess, she thought. There were malfunctions everywhere. She focused on the speed. Could she believe it? It was true. They had hit light speed. She glared at what hitherto should have been an impossible figure, then noticed that the figure was still increasing at a gradual rate. Impossible . . . impossible . . . she thought.

Similar mayhem was being re-enacted all over the craft as the crew struggled to come to grips with the situation. Communications became impossible in the sense that they suffered from the same one way directional problems as did vision. Maria, with eyes ablaze and mouth open, determined that acceleration was still occurring and the speed still edging upwards. Then there was another shock, this time a more pleasant one at least.

Without any warning, the darkness receded as rapidly as it had arrived. Adam and Maria turned, open-mouthed, and faced each other. They disentangled their linked arms; an embrace seemed far more appropriate. Adam quickly broke from Maria's arms, albeit reluctantly, and turned his attention to the displays in front of him. There a mass of flashing gobbledygook met his eyes. His hands moved forward, but Maria grasped them.

'No, don't touch anything,' she hissed uncharacteristically.

'But . . .'

'No ... No ... Whatever has happened, it's under control, or at least stable ...' Maria's voice tailed off, realising that probably her choice of words could have been better, but the thought of anything being touched and reproducing the darkness was her major concern. Adam caught the meaning in her statement, however, and withdrew his hands as if he had touched a hotplate.

'You're right, of course. Let's get everyone together first and do some reassuring, then we'll plan what to do after that.'

Adam's mind whirled. The whole enterprise had been so carefully planned and life on board the DSP so predictable. No one had seriously expected any major problems. Now a real test of their skills confronted them, and it would take every fibre of their wits to unravel the predicament.

The intercoms sprang back to two way communication once 'the black,' as the crew would subsequently refer to it, subsided. Adam sent an immediate assembly message. The crew buzzed with an excitement, stimulated by a mixture of fear, elation and anticipation. Adam bustled to the front and a spontaneous hush overcame his audience. He sounded breathless as he spoke.

'Something has propelled us past light speed. I take it you all suffered the same one way vision that Maria and I did.'

The murmuring and nodding confirmed that everyone had. David and Anna had been together and not had the benefit of any technical information when the phenomenon occurred. David was dumbfounded and glared at Anna as he recalled her prophetic theorising earlier. Anna swallowed hard, making a gulping noise as she did so. She vowed never to make smart remarks about science again ... as long as she lived. Not that, as things currently appeared, that would be very long.

Meanwhile, Adam continued, 'Our next task is to analyse things as quickly as possible and see what steps we should take.'

He looked about the sea of faces in front of him. 'Jack?'

'Here, Cap.'

'Are your displays full of malfunctions?'

'They sure are Cap. But don't worry. It may be merely a matter of resetting them to see what is really going on.'

Jack's sober answer reassured Adam. Combined with Maria's earlier stoicism it generated pride in his crew. In the meantime Jack continued, 'We should have recordings of the events, so we'll study them and see what we've got.'

A few of the crew had suffered minor injuries, including Henny, who sported a large blister on the back of her right hand. These were directed to the medical team, the rest into functional groups, as a form of damage control. Adam and his co-commanders gathered up Jack and hastened to the command centre. Jack left Bud to stand by in the main computer area. Jack isolated the recordings that Adam and his group longed to study. He and Alex then began to reproduce them stepwise as the others watched intently.

'That's it . . . stop there . . . that's where it happened,' snapped Yvonne, 'I felt it . . .'

'Just as I was about to pause acceleration,' said Adam ruefully.

'Don't worry, Cap,' said Jack with a grin, 'we seem to have survived it all. I think we will be patting ourselves on the back in due course.'

'I admire your optimism, Jack, but it's a bit soon for the patting, as you call it. I don't think that my heart will stop racing for a month!'

'Here come all the errors and malfunctions,' continued Jack, as he flicked on the next phase of the recorded data. he stopped the sequence and they all studied the screen.

'Anyone see a pattern?' asked Jack in a tone that

intimated that he already knew the answer.

Alex provided it. 'Yes. The malfunctions consist of true malfunctions and what the computer regards as "errors".'

'There's a difference?' questioned Adam.

'Yes, Cap. A malfunction means that something broke down, whereas an error means that the computer has decided that an item is inappropriate.'

Adam still wasn't quite sure that he fully understood the subtle difference, but his scientific colleagues were nodding assent, obviously indicating that they did. Jack explained further, clarifying the situation for Adam.

'All the malfunctions have been caused by transmission failures by fibre optics, presumably as a result of the forward failure that we had.'

'So what do we do?' asked Adam.

'I'll round up my techs and have the problem fixed in no time,' came Jack's reply.

'And the errors?'

'That's for your brains trust here to figure out,' said Jack with a grin. 'It looks like you'll have to come up with a few new time and motion laws . . .'

On that mischievous note Jack departed.

'Well, Brains Trust? . . . ' said Adam, managing his first smile since their predicament began.

'We'll do some reprogramming, so that the computers accept the current state of affairs . . . whatever they may be . . .' said Maria.

The crew worked feverishly for the next hour. Those not directly involved in immediate technical duties were dispatched on reconnaissance missions to directly inspect the more remote sections of the craft. Carl and Tony assessed the state of the all-important food supply, and were joined in due course by Anna. Fortunately there appeared to be no immediate problems. Bud and a band of helpers had disappeared into the rear of the DSP to make a direct inspection of the rear engines and reactors. En route they turned off various alarms and reset much in the way of faulty mechanisms such as remote communications, emergency door locks and other basic functions. These activities proved much more time-consuming than those performed by the senior members of the crew. In fact Jack, along with Maria, had their reprogramming completed as predicted within the hour.

Adam surveyed the displays which now had ceased their blinking and had returned to an orderly format.

'I suppose what's on the screen is true information,' he said. 'I find it hard to believe that velocity, though.'

'How can it be?' added Alex. The intercom prevented him from elaborating further. Anna's face appeared.

'Anna!' exclaimed Adam. 'Everything OK?'

'Yes, Captain. Is it convenient for me to come up?'

Adam frowned. Why was everyone calling him 'Captain' all of a sudden? The formality had been rarely used on the mission until now.

'Yes, by all means come.'

'I don't think it's very important. It's David's idea that I should see you. It's silly really . . .'

'Come on up,' interrupted Adam, deciding that if David had made the suggestion, then Anna must have something significant to discuss.

Anna appeared within minutes and stood rather starchily to attention.

'For goodness sake, Anna, sit down. In fact let's all relax for a few minutes, and why is everyone calling me Captain?'

Anna grinned at the request for an answer to this piece of trivia and composed herself. 'Well, Cap . . . er, Adam, I think that we are all feeling a trifle insecure and we're looking to our leader for hope and guidance.'

Adam stared at Anna with a quizzical expression, the

weight of responsibility and the fate of his crew suddenly emerging from his subconscious mind. In the meantime Maria said, 'We're dying to know what you've come about, Anna, or is it confidential?'

'No definitely not, except you will think that I'm wasting your time. I had this stupid conversation with David before the . . . well, whatever it was that happened. You know, I had been voicing my insecurities about the approach to light speed.'

'Yes, I remember our conversation,' said Maria, 'perhaps I should have taken you more seriously!'

'No . . . I was just being silly really. Anyway I was poking a bit of fun at David about passing the speed of light being not much different to passing the speed of sound.'

'You were no doubt thinking about all the doom and gloom predicted for the individuals in the mid-twentieth century who contemplated breaking the so-called sound barrier,' said Alex.

'Yes . . . it's a bit of a habit of mine, I'm afraid, to poke fun at pompous scientists who have had their pet theories overturned. Er . . . nothing against present company of course,' added Anna hastily.

Yvonne laughed and replied, 'I think we are more the crazy, adventurous type scientists, rather than the pompous type. Why, look at Maria. She used to defy the law of gravity with her leaps and somersaults!'

'I'm glad you said "used to". I'm a bit past that sort of thing now,' said Maria.

Alex brought the discussion back to the point. 'Anna, tell us more about your theories.'

'I don't think they deserve to be called theories,' said Anna modestly, 'more like wild guesses. However, as I see it, the speed of sound is a finite number and can be passed. Likewise the speed of light is a finite number, albeit a much larger one, so I don't see why that can't be exceeded as well.'

Adam cast his eyes around his scientific colleagues and said, 'Am I right in saying that the velocities greater than the speed of light contradict the formulae?'

Jack, who had been silent, entered the conversation. 'Perhaps our formulae are only valid up to the speed of light . . . just as Newton's formulae are only valid up to a certain point.'

Jack smiled with satisfaction; he also enjoyed playing devil's advocate.

'Of course you are right,' answered Alex surprisingly. 'As usual we do not look beyond the ends of our noses. No one has bothered to consider the situation of an object travelling faster than the speed of light. It is like those who considered that the Sun revolved around the Earth. No one considered it. The facts had to be gathered in a practical manner by Galileo and his telescope.'

The hitherto sober discussion suddenly burst to life. Yvonne gave a whoop. 'Anna, you're a genius. Trust a doctor to hand us a diagnosis!'

'Diagnosis?'

'Yes . . . yes . . . Why shouldn't we travel as fast as we like? Just because stupid photons can't travel any faster . . .'

'You seem to be forgetting that they must be travelling faster now; otherwise half of us would be in the dark, like we were earlier,' said Alex.

'Something flips at light speed . . . that's for sure,' said Maria with a frown.

Jack spoke again.'I guess the relativity formulae are obsolete.'

The remark drew a sharp look from the scientists, as if a great heresy had been pronounced.

'The point,' said Alex, 'is that relativity is supposed to cater for all situations.'

'Well it's been around for a long time,' said Jack, 'we'd better come up with something new.'

Adam turned to more practical matters. 'This intellectual discussion is all very fascinating, I'm sure, but will you nouveaux Einsteins like to tell me where this all leaves us?'

Jack answered immediately. 'Well, Cap, we're travelling at 1.5c and before all hell broke loose our trajectory was aimed at Proxima Centauri. Our guidance froze when all the malfunctions lit up, so we should be on the same flight path. Yet according to all the data in front of you, we are pointing at blank space!'

Adam thought for a minute, then said, 'I still don't understand what could have caused this . . .'

'I think I can offer an explanation,' said Maria. The others turned to her, eager to hear it.

'As you know, something propelled us forward at an incredible rate. It wasn't our own power, so it must have been something behind us.'

'You mean something gave us a giant kick in the pants . . . but what?' questioned Adam.

'Our emissions . . .'

'Our emissions . . . how?' asked Adam before anyone else could speak.

'Well, put simply, our mass approaches infinity near light speed, but in here it is all fairly meaningless as the forces are balanced, so to speak. However, particles flung out of the engines would have been objects of infinite mass being flung against each other in a completely disordered manner. The result was almost certainly a huge nuclear reaction. We probably only escaped complete annihilation by the skin of our teeth because we were travelling so fast that we outran it . . . just!'

'And we wouldn't feel the acceleration, as we weren't in a gravitational field,' added Yvonne, 'yet I thought I noticed something . . . it was barely perceptible.'

‘Possibly a faint pull from the rear,’ said Alex, eager to make a further contribution to the conversation.

Adam turned to Anna. ‘Our joke about the oranges, it had a grain of reality, Anna . . .’

Anna just smiled. Adam continued, ‘What will they receive back on Earth, I wonder?’

‘No doubt they will see a giant explosion,’ said Alex with a frown.

Adam spun to the console behind him. Yvonne read his thoughts. ‘It’s no good transmitting Adam, the signal won’t escape our forward velocity.’

Anna gasped, ‘Joe, what will they do to Joe?’

‘They will assume that the DSP has gone up in smoke and us along with it,’ said Alex forlornly, ‘. . . they’ll crucify him!’

7

'Great! Just great!' blustered Adam. 'We're beetling along, for all practical purposes out of control, and with no sense of direction and we don't know what to do about it!'

He glared at his senior colleagues, frustrated at their inability to produce a solution to their predicament. Seventy two hours had passed since the catastrophe and the 'brains trust' were no closer to a solution than when the event first took place. Adam composed himself and then modified his tone in response to the uncharacteristically drawn expressions which faced him. He was aware that they, like himself, had hardly slept whilst they agonised over their problems.

'Well . . . we have to do something. We can't fly like this forever. Otherwise we'll end up in deep space and run out of supplies.'

'Nothing adds up,' said Alex in frustration. 'We can't make any calculations if we can't fathom out the laws which are governing our motion.'

'Why can't we just slow down?' said Adam, waving his arms about.

'Because if Maria is right about the explosion at light speed, caused by particles of infinite mass, if we fire retrothrust we'll fly right into the fire, so to speak,' answered Alex.

'What about the small guidance rockets which are offset

from the main craft?' said Adam hopefully.

'I thought of that,' Maria said with a sigh. 'Unfortunately, as we slowed we'd be in range of the explosion, if it occurred.'

'What do you mean — if it occurred?'

'Well it doesn't necessarily follow that the same phenomenon occurs in reverse. I mean, compare it with the sonic booms when the sound barrier is broken. They don't reoccur when one slows down again.'

'A good point, Maria,' said Alex, sounding impressed, 'but you must agree we can hardly put it to the test.'

Adam rather hoped that Maria might reply with a feasible answer, but a frown was the only response that the exhausted mathematician could manage.

'Something must be happening with time,' said Yvonne, changing the thrust of the conversation. 'It's the only way that our equations will make sense.'

'So what do we do?' said Adam pointedly, bringing the conversation back to more practical matters.

'I hate to say it, Adam, but until we can come up with some answers I don't think that we should do anything.'

Yvonne immediately noticed the colour rise in Adam's face and spoke quickly to relieve his frustration. 'Adam, I know it all seems impossible and out of control at present, but obviously we are capable of great speeds at least. It is a matter of turning this new-found power to our advantage.'

'And in the meantime . . .?'

'Do no harm, leave things alone,' said Maria.

'Exactly!' Yvonne concurred.

Adam flopped back, exhausted. 'So my only consolation is that if we do nothing, at least things won't get worse.'

Three heads nodded apologetically in reply. Frustration and depression, fuelled by mental and physical fatigue, began to overtake the scientists. An adjournment was decided upon and they returned to their quarters, leaving Adam to brood alone in the command centre.

Jack and his technicians experienced no such frustrations. Within the realms of the craft they had virtually everything working perfectly. Jack had made intermittent contact with Adam, though, and was well aware of his problems. In amongst their duties the technicians had also debated their predicament. Jack held his own mini-conference with his two immediate subordinates, Bud and Helen.

'Sooner or later they'll want the engines on line again,' said Jack, 'so we'd better send a team to the front and rear.'

'Do we really need to worry about the rear at this stage?' said Bud. 'We'll be unlikely to be using any forward thrust for a bit.'

'I'm a bit concerned about what might have happened as a result of this supposed explosion. I think everything should be checked, including all the operating programs at the reactor.'

'Fair enough,' replied Bud, 'that's quite a bit of work!'

'Yes, I know, think you can handle it? With some assistance, of course.'

'My pleasure,' said Bud with a grin, 'who do I get for company?'

'Well, as you say, it is a big job. Normally I'd say the lot of us, but I can probably do the front end with one or two. It will be more or less routine.'

'Why not use Kate?' said Helen. 'She spends more time helping us than she does nursing, and she's really good.'

'Yes, good suggestion. I'm sure Loretta can hold the fort if there's an outbreak of measles,' replied Jack with a grin. 'Very well, Bud, I'll take Bernard and Kate. You can have the rest. Between you and Helen you shouldn't have any problems. OK with you, Helen?'

'Fine,' said Helen. 'I'm looking forward to doing something constructive.'

'It'll be more like tedium and boredom,' said Bud, noticing Jack nodding in agreement, 'but it will help pass the time whilst the clever dicks come up with some answers.'

'I'd better let Adam know what we're up to,' said Jack as he accessed the intercom. Adam's weary face appeared. Jack outlined their plans, and Adam appeared pleased that someone was doing something constructive.

'I shouldn't be away too long, Cap,' said Jack in conclusion. 'The craft is running like clockwork, internally anyway, so if there's any problem give me a buzz and I'll come straight back.'

Bud and Helen rounded up Carmel, Alan and Stephanie. They stopped by the catering area and collected some supplies from Henny and then set off to the rear of the craft.

Bud and his group drifted weightlessly into the cavernous area which contained the 'brains' of the reactors and the main engines. Computer terminals ringed the area. A circular bar, designed to steady the operators of the terminals in a weightless environment also encircled the area. The five techs initially gathered near the main control unit which virtually duplicated its counterpart in the command centre. Bud brought the display to life and switched it to off line.

'We'll grab a terminal each, and if everyone can go through stepwise and then verify with either Helen or myself.'

The group nodded in response to Bud's directive and drifted into their respective positions. Bud called after them, 'Check reactor status first, then we'll set it up for prefunctional operation.'

The task proved much more laborious than they had expected. Everything had shut down automatically, but not before a Pandora's box of error readings had infected the programming. Bud and Helen struggled, as they had to start from scratch. Apart from this the restraining bar had obviously been designed for larger individuals. Helen found that she could not brace herself effectively and kept flying off the keyboard. She eventually looked across to see how the others had come to terms with the problem. Carmel, who was slightly taller than Helen, just managed to reach the bar with her bottom, though she had to extend her arms fully forward, the overall line of her body looking quite seductive, Stephanie, who was easily the shortest, simply wrapped her knees around the bar trapeze style and lay horizontally, leaving her hands in near perfect position. Neither of these two positions appeared to suit Helen. At last she worked out a composite position with one foot against the bar and her left hand counterbalancing on the console. This left her to operate the keyboard with her remaining hand.

'This area was designed for Amazons,' she muttered. However, the group soon became much too absorbed to worry about the contortions of each other's bodies.

Several hours passed before Bud called for a halt. 'Let's have a rest . . . and something to eat.'

The others sighed with approval and drifted off into the centre. Despite the climate control, they felt quite hot and stripped down to T-shirts, with the exception of Stephanie who didn't seem to notice the warmth as much as the others, though she appeared quite flushed.

Another twelve hours would pass before Bud's group would complete their task. At the end they were quite exhausted and hung like washing on a clothes line in the middle of the room, tired and hungry again. The task had demanded so much concentration that they all felt even more hot and bothered, Helen had unashamedly removed her slacks and sneakers and had worked for the last few hours in T-shirt and knickers. Bud and Alan were topless and Carmel had exposed her midriff. Only Stephanie had remained fully clad, though she had pulled up her sleeves and removed her shoes. The discarded items of clothing were lined up in mid-air in comical fashion to provide some light-hearted humour, counterbalancing the otherwise serious task.

'Well . . . finished at last,' said Bud. 'All I have to do is reconnect this area with the bridge.'

He returned to the main console and typed in the appropriate commands. When operational, the rear engines were virtually silent. However, there was no mistaking the fact that they had come to life. Helen, who had just put her feet into her slacks, spun around and spoke the words that the others were thinking.

'Bud . . . the engines . . . we're accelerating, what . . .?'

Bud stiffened and replied, 'Quick everyone check, all I did was reconnect with the bridge I'm sure . . .!'

The five returned to the displays, which quickly confirmed that everything was as it should be.

Jack had joined Adam sometime previously, his task at the front of the craft long completed. He had managed to divert Adam's attention away from the immediate problems of the DSP by recounting some of his experiences in the naval reserve. Adam's attention was suddenly diverted by a change of status, which was automatically displayed on the screen in front of him. Simultaneously, Bud appeared on the intercom.

'Adam . . . we're accelerating!'

'I know . . . at least I've just noticed ... how do you know?'

'I'm in the rear engine chamber, we've just finished. I swear I didn't start anything. That can only be done from the bridge anyway.'

'I didn't touch a thing!' replied Adam with the air of a child who has been caught in the act of some misdemeanour. The normally unruffable Jack gasped as he surveyed the display in more detail.

'Cap, not only are we accelerating, but at an incredible rate!'

Adam was dumbfounded. Meanwhile Jack took over the conversation with Bud. 'Bud when did the engines restart?'

'As far as I can tell, when I reconnected the engine room with the bridge, I . . .'

'Hang on Bud,' interrupted Jack. He turned to Adam.

'Adam do you remember the status of the engines when we had our "big bang" or whatever . . .?'

'They were programmed to shut down automatically . . . which I presume they did . . .'

Jack turned again to Bud's image and said, 'Bud what was the initial status of the engines?'

'No status. There were errors all over the place which presumably resulted in them shutting down.'

'That's it!' snapped Jack. 'Adam, the engines stopped due to local systems failure, not due to a command from here which was never received. Now that they're reconnected, your old command has been revalidated.'

'So it should be a simple matter to turn them off,' said Adam, quickly grasping the situation.

Jack watched intently as Adam gave the command to shut down the engines.

'Are they off?' he asked Bud.

'Off . . . confirmed,' came Bud's immediate reply. 'What's our speed according to you, Jack?'

'About ten times light speed,' gulped Jack.

'Same reading here,' said Bud, 'yet the engines couldn't have been on for even a full minute!'

'So a little thrust produces a large effect. Thanks Bud, are you all finished?'

'Yes, we were preparing to come back.'

'Very well, tell the others to take a break. You as well, I'll be in touch later.'

Jack turned to Adam. 'Cap . . . we may have accidently stumbled onto some answers . . .'

'What do you mean?'

'I suggest you get Maria up here, with the empirical data from the engine burn. Her clever mind should be able to come up with a new motion equation.'

Maria had obviously been awoken from a deep sleep. Normally she was well groomed and was one of the few crew members to wear the 'uniform' of the DSP. But then with her figure she was one of the few that managed to still appear attractive in it. With the urgency of the situation, however, she had thrown on a pair of shorts and a loose-fitting top. She flicked her hair off her face as she hastened to the command centre. Adam and Jack hardly recognised the figure who hurried towards them. Their blank faces drew a quizzical response from Maria. 'What is it? You said it was urgent.'

'We accidently activated the engines,' said Adam, not wanting to go into too much detail, 'Jack will explain.'

'Bud restored the engine room communications with the bridge,' continued Jack. 'It appears that they had shut themselves down due to malfunction, so that when they were reconnected to here, they just obeyed the previous commands prior to the black out.'

Maria's quick mind grasped the situation without need for any further explanation, she studied the display and exclaimed. 'Good Lord! Ten times light speed. How long did you leave the engines on?'

'That's the point,' broke in Adam, 'it was less than a minute.'

Jack smiled as he sensed Maria coming to same conclusions he had. He didn't speak. Instead he allowed her the satisfaction of voicing the conclusion herself.

'So . . . small burn . . . big response . . . Of course, why didn't we think of it before? We're fools!'

'We are?' said Adam.

'Of course!' continued Maria. 'We were that paranoid about not touching anything, in particular not slowing down. We thought the only way to solve our problems was by theoretical means. This incident should give us the information that we need to devise a formula.'

'Atta girl,' said Jack with a big smile.

Maria flopped back, once again pushing her unruly hair off her face.

'I still can't believe how stupid we were . . . Adam, you tried to get us to do something and we all behaved like nervous Nellies. If we were so scared of slowing down, all we had to do was speed up a bit, gather the information, stop, then draw our conclusions, and then worry about slowing down.'

'I don't know that I would have been all that keen on speeding up further,' admitted Adam.

'Can we get the others?' asked Maria, 'they should be in on this.'

Although interested in the conclusion, Jack decided that he had contributed enough to the discussion and excused himself. Alex and Yvonne appeared soon after and were soon acquainted with the latest developments. Together, with Adam and Maria, they poured over the information provided by the accidental engine burn. It took about one hour before they drew their conclusions.

'According to our figures, it's as Maria says. Each small increase in thrust increases our velocity at an exponential rate,' said Alex.

Maria had been somewhat silent, her brain obviously in overdrive. She had the slight advantage over the others of having had longer to mull over the data. She suddenly leapt to her feet, grasping the waist of her shorts and hitching them up, almost as if she expected the revelation which she was about to make, might cause them to fall down.

'It flip . . . inverts . . . oh! What do you call it?' she said in frustration, at first unable to explain herself. No prompting came, however, from the others. Eventually she managed to articulate what she meant. 'Ooh . . . time . . . it becomes negative beyond the speed of light.'

Alex and Yvonne's minds immediately tuned to Maria's, as if telepathic. Yvonne just managed to speak before Alex. 'Yes . . . yes . . . it explains everything perfectly, it's a sudden change. Then as velocity increases, our mass decreases. Therefore thrust has an ever increasing effect, just as was demonstrated with the accidental firing of the engines.'

The scientists were clearly elated beyond description. In Adam's estimation it would be another half hour before they were to speak sense again. They kept repeating the same conclusions over and over again, like a group of sports fans recounting their team's winning moment. Eventually they all stumbled over each other in their attempts to explain the situation to Adam, but from his perception it was all confused gobbledygook. He nodded politely and repeatedly mouthed. 'I see.' But he was really none the wiser at the conclusion of the explanations. 'As usual no one offers me any practical advice', he thought. Eventually the hubbub subsided.

'Er . . . Maria . . .' said Adam, 'can you come with me to see Jack about a few things? Alex, can you take over on the bridge for a bit?'

Alex, Maria and Yvonne looked at Adam as if he were some spoiled sport who was breaking up their birthday party half an hour after it had commenced. Adam read their thoughts.

'Don't worry, you lot, you can get together later and talk till the cows come home. But there are a few practical matters I wish to sort out.'

The scientists nodded, puzzled that anyone would be interested in anything other than their new discovery.

Maria linked her arm with Adam's as they proceeded down the corridor. A satisfied smile dominated her expression. She looked altogether out of character in her attire as she flounced along, almost breaking into a skip at times. Her soft breast continually assaulted Adam's left arm, which induced a satisfied expression on his face. The human warmth from his companion compensated for the tensions of the previous few days. Their somewhat uncharacteristic appearance raised Jack's eyebrows as they arrived unannounced.

'You look like you've just won the lottery,' quipped Jack.

'We have, we have,' answered Maria.

'OK, Miss Enthusiasm . . . before you get too carried away, you may as well know that I haven't a clue what you were raving about up there,' said Adam.

'We did get rather carried away, didn't we? But it's so exciting . . .'

'Tell us in words of one syllable then,' said Jack.

'Very well . . .' said Maria drawing a deep breath. 'You understand that as we approach the speed of light we approach infinite mass.'

'Yes, we understand,' said Adam, thinking that if he heard that statement one more time he would go crazy.

'Yes . . . well . . . for the mass equation to stay real beyond the speed of light, time must become negative.'

'Time squared,' interrupted Jack.

'Time squared?'

'Yes, lass. Negative time would be squared in your mass equation so it would remain unreal.'

Maria looked completely deflated. Adam retained his continued state of bewilderment. 'Our marvellous theory . . . it's incorrect . . . yet it explains things. How could I have overlooked . . .'

'Oh, your conclusions are correct my girl. In fact it's our distance . . . Distance squared at least which is negative, but then that is interrelated with time, it seems. The conclusion is the same.'

'I came down here to clear things up,' interjected Adam. 'Now I'm more confused than ever.'

Maria became a picture of concentration.

'I'm getting the picture Jack,' she said, 'how did you figure it out?'

'I didn't. Someone left me a note,' replied Jack and handed a piece of paper to Maria. She studied it intently.

'Time travel!' she exclaimed and lapsed back into intense concentration. Adam looked searchingly at Jack who merely shrugged his shoulders in response. Meanwhile Maria had deposited herself on the floor and appeared hypnotised by the contents of the note. Adam knew it would be useless to interrupt her; she would speak when ready.

Maria eventually raised her eyes. 'This is brillaint . . . who wrote it?'

'I've no idea . . . it was left under my door.'

'Care to share your thoughts?' asked Adam.

Maria spoke carefully as she replied, 'Well . . . we are familiar with our own time reference and the universe as we see it. So we've framed our laws accordingly and the movement of the universe around us conforms. It's a bit like the state of affairs when people looked up in the sky and assumed that the Sun was rotating around the Earth. It was a reasonable conclusion, given the facts as they could see them. If they had shot themselves into a different dimension, say into space, they would have discovered a different dimension to the immediate universe as they knew it. They couldn't travel into space of course, but Galileo did, indirectly, with his telescope and found the answers.'

Adam and Jack remained silent; at last things appeared to be making sense, so they didn't dare interrupt. Maria continued, 'We have moved out of our dimension again, which is apparently bounded by the speed of light. The universe, it seems, has its own fundamental time scale or movement or displacement along an absolute time scale and we are crossing it.'

Maria fell silent. Adam waited a minute and then said, 'Anything else?'

'Yes. Who is the genius who wrote this note?' she replied with a wry smile.

Jack grinned. 'I've no idea, as you can see from the ending, someone who doesn't "wish to make a big deal" out of it.'

'What does this mean in practical terms?' asked Adam.

'Well the universe is moving in space along some sort of axis. What we are familiar with, of course, is movement "within" the universe itself. It's like being on the surface of the Earth. We are aware of local movements, for example running, driving or flying around, but we aren't aware that the Earth is whizzing through space around the Sun.'

'I think I'm finally beginning to comprehend,' said Adam. Maria extended her arm towards Adam, apparently hoping he would help her off the floor. He responded to the gesture and pulled her up. She gave an exhuberant hop and straightened herself out. She smiled at Adam, then turned to Jack.

'If we obtain some reference points, Jack, we can possibly calculate at what angle to the displacement axis of the universe we are flying.'

'That could be difficult at this speed.' replied Jack, 'but we can try.'

'What did you mean about time travel?' said Adam.

'Well . . . If we can fly along the very axis of the universe at any speed we like, then we can literally visit any point in space or time that we like, at least theoretically. It might take something a bit more sophisticated than this tub, though.'

'If we've discovered time travel, then it's likely others have, I mean from other star systems,' said Adam.

'Or it's possible that we bring the discovery back to Earth and it's utilised,' added Jack, 'but does that mean that we can go back in time and change things?'

'I shouldn't think so,' said Maria, 'for example . . . if you went back to assassinate Hitler or someone like that, you'd fail, we know that. But there may be things done by time travellers that we are unaware of. Or events caused by them. Only we didn't realise that they did them. If you travel back in time, it would be like travelling anywhere else . . . you take your chances.'

'So the UFO sightings may be real after all,' said Adam.

'Some of them, anyway,' replied Maria.

8

'Outside!' exclaimed Adam, 'but it could be dangerous!'

'I don't see how conditions out there should be any different to in here, Cap,' said Jack reassuringly.

'We don't have much choice, Adam, we need a remote drive source. It will be easy enough to construct inside. Then it is just a matter of attaching it and connecting it up,' added Alex.

'It will be fairly routine exterior work, Cap,' said Jack.

'Very well,' said Adam, 'what exactly are the details?'

'We need a very fine drive force. An ion gun would be the simplest, as our main drive is far too powerful under these conditions; even our manipulator and docking jets are way too powerful. Also, if we are concerned about braking near light speed, then ions will be far safer,' said Yvonne.

'Jack, how will you go about it?' asked Adam.

'We can assemble most of it in the bay. It will be relatively straightforward in the weightless area. Then we'll float it out and attach it.'

In spite of the reassurances, Adam still wore a concerned expression. He continued, 'Who goes outside then?'

'Well, I would . . .'

'No . . . not you,' interrupted Adam, 'I can't take risks with senior personnel!'

Jack shrugged his shoulders. Alex studied Adam intently.

He knew that Adam had not taken any worthwhile rest for days and he could tell that the stress was beginning to take its toll. Eventually Jack said, 'I can send Bud, Cap, but I don't regard the procedure as risky, and I was thinking more along the lines that it will be even safer if properly supervised.'

'Bud is reliable?'

'Very reliable,' answered Jack, feeling slighted that one of his techs should be thought of in any other way.

'Who else?'

'Well, ideally the more the better, but I guess you wouldn't approve of everyone going.' A note of sarcasm had crept into the normally jovial senior technician's voice.

'No. Only half of them at the most.'

Alex felt the need to speak in support of Jack. 'Adam, you're talking as if you're expecting them not to return.'

Adam drew a long breath. He was aware of his slightly belligerent attitude, which he could not control in his present state of mind. However, he had his reasons for the caution he was displaying. He chose his next words carefully and spoke as a captain would.

'The whole point of the exercise that you have suggested is to provide us with fine tuning to our movements . . . correct?'

'Correct,' replied Alex.

'So, if in achieving these fine movements we lose control, or there are any accidents which displace personnel from the immediate vicinity of the craft, then we can't exactly go after them . . . can we!'

Jack answered for the group. 'Point taken, Cap, I guess that's why you're the Captain and we're the crew.'

The remark lightened the mood and everyone relaxed.

'Realistically Jack, can four of the techs do the job?' asked Adam.

'Yes, Cap, it'll take a while longer of course.'

'Very well, it's settled. Who will you send?'

Jack thought for a minute. Bud, of course, would lead, but Adam's fear of danger and even the unthinkable loss of members of his team made it difficult for him to decide between youth or experience. Eventually he answered, 'Apart from Bud, I'll send Alan and . . . Carmel and Stephanie . . . they're the least experienced, but extremely competent.'

And dispensible, thought Yvonne with a shudder. Poor Jack, being put in such a position, but really . . . what could go wrong?

The meeting broke up. Maria had been silent during the latter discussions. She had earlier given a discourse on her 'absolute universal time' conclusions which had, in turn, sparked the discussion on the control of the DSP's motion. She now walked back towards the quarters with Yvonne.

'Let's hope there aren't any space monsters out there.'

Yvonne managed a smile, before replying, 'Something has got Adam worried. I hope the space walkers don't pick up the vibes.'

'How well do you know the two girls?' asked Maria.

'Hardly at all . . . At least I've worked with Carmel briefly on occasions; she's very bright and outgoing. Stephanie keeps to herself mainly; Jack is very protective towards her. I believe that she was the last one selected for the mission.'

'Let's hope she's not . . .'

'Don't . . .' interrupted Yvonne. 'Why has everyone become infected with doom and gloom?'

'I'm sorry,' said Maria, 'it must be the let down after the excitement of our new discoveries.'

Maria felt a strange premonition, however, and try as she would, she found it difficult to banish it from her mind.

Jack faced Bud, Alan, Carmel and Stephanie.

'We need to construct an ion gun to control our fine movements. The assembly will be done in the bay, but I've chosen you four to take it out and attach it.'

Four pairs of eyes widened.

'You're not coming, Jack?' said Bud.

'I thought you'd enjoy the adventure more.' Jack replied, concealing the true reason.

'I suppose Adam doesn't want to risk losing his chief technician,' said Bud with a laugh.

'I don't expect anyone to be lost . . .'

'Just joking, Jack, you know how cautious I am. We'll take care, won't we, team?'

'It'll sure beat waste treatment duties,' replied Carmel, referring to the bane of the techs' lives on board the DSP.

Jack cast his eyes along the group. They rested momentarily on Stephanie, who smiled, as if to reassure him. He then turned his head and continued.

'OK, we'll all assist with the assembly initially. I suggest all you four don exterior suits for the final stages, so that you can get the hang of working in them before going out.'

Whilst the techs busied themselves on the assembly of the new power source, David paid a visit to the command centre. Whatever the demands of their predicament, he had decided to make some recommendations.

'The crew has to be rested Adam, and that includes you.'

Adam glared at David's solemn expression and replied, 'I don't think that you realise the seriousness of the situation. We have got to regain control before we are lost forever . . . and you want us to rest!'

'Making the wrong decisions due to fatigue won't help us,' retorted David.

The firmness of David's tone was unfamiliar to Adam. He responded with equal conviction. 'Listen, David, I'm in charge and I will decide . . .'

'We need a plan,' interrupted David.

'A plan? What sort of plan?'

'A plan to rest the crew,' continued David. 'I don't mean all at once, but in waves or whatever.'

'I know what you mean,' said Adam, softening his tone a little, 'but it won't be that easy.'

'But surely it's just a matter of more or less dividing each division in half and sending half to rest.'

'Unfortunately the techs, as you know, are the lifeblood of this craft ... even more so now. In fact they're all engaged at present and soon half of them will be going outside,' came Adam's reply.

'Outside!' exclaimed David. 'Good grief, what for?'

Adam explained the need for the offset power source. David thought for a minute but continued with his original mission.

'Very well. I'll start at the top. Adam, you're a walking zombie, so how about handing over?'

Adam began to speak but David promptly stifled the response. 'No ifs or buts, Captain, I know full well your value in keeping morale high, but sooner or later you'll have to give the co-commanders a turn.'

Whilst David cajoled his captain off the bridge, the techs were at work in the cavernous docking area, assembling the superstructure which would be required to carry the new power source. The weightless environment made the task relatively straightforward. For the latter stages of the procedure, the four chosen to spacewalk donned their exterior suits for the sake of familiarisation. Helen participated in the dress-up, as Jack and Bud had decided that she would remain in the bay, when depressurised, to assist. Even though Adam had limited the number of spacewalkers to four, Jack had determined that Helen, for practical purposes, would still be 'inside.' He hoped that Adam would understand the liberal interpretation of the original command.

Although 'climate controlled', those working in the suits became quite hot as their movements were grossly restricted. Eventually the final stages were completed. Helen struggled out of her suit, wet with perspiration.

'Phew ... I don't envy you lot working out there for any length of time,' she remarked as she noticed the equally red faces before her.

'You're right,' replied Bud, 'a simple task sure becomes complicated when you're trussed up in a suit.'

They stripped down to underwear and hung in midair. Loretta, who had joined the group as an observer, disappeared briefly and returned with a handful of towels to mop the fevered brows. Duly rested, Bud, Carmel, Alan and Stephanie prepared for their new adventure. Helen also prepared for her auxiliary role.

Jack closed the air lock and, the task completed, the giant exterior doors of the bay unfolded to reveal an enormous expanse of pitch blackness. Stephanie shuddered slightly as she stared into the void which would shortly devour them. She bit her already dry lower lip and drew a deep breath. As she exhaled Bud's voice filled her helmet: 'OK team ... in line.'

The four adopted their pre-arranged positions as Helen swam beneath the large gantry in readiness to push it out of the bay. A feeling of omnipotence enveloped her as she pushed the structure into motion. Her colleagues were dotted about it symmetrically in order to control its motion. Each held small hand jets to control themselves and the positioning of their giant piece of apparatus. They also wore line guns which they could fire at the body of the DSP to secure themselves in an emergency; otherwise they floated free in the vacuum of deep space. The operation began smoothly enough, though predictably the team members once again found their suits restrictive and cumbersome. Bud conducted his players like a master of ceremonies.

With coordinated firing of their jets they drifted towards the rear of the craft. External lighting picked them out like bright dots against the total void around them, though occasionally when looking in the direct line of their motion, they thought that they could see transient flashes ahead. The eeriness struck all four and Bud kept up a constant banter to maintain the morale of the group. All had been outside before, but usually with the bright globe of the Earth or Moon about them and with the heavens sparkling in the distance. Now they were in total darkness except for the light that they provided for themselves, either on their suits or from the main body of the DSP. Having arrived at their arranged position, they set to work near the rear of the craft. Helen sneaked up to the edge of the docking bay and watched from a distance.

They had anticipated one to two hours for the assembly, but after two hours only fifty per cent of the operation had been completed. Bud called a halt and the group returned to the bay. Once inside, the area was repressurised and the four, plus Helen, extricated themselves from the confines of the suits. The semi-naked parade turned as Jack entered the chamber. Carmel swept her sodden hair off her face and flicked her head so that her luxuriant locks fanned out behind her.

'You look like you would enjoy a swim in a nice cool river,' said Helen with a grin.

Stephanie moved up next to them. She wore the excited expression of a child that has just survived her first ride on a roller coaster. She was clad in a loose T-shirt, distended in the front by the mounds of her prominent breasts and a brief pair of knickers. Even so she was considerably better attired than her colleagues, who had decided that they would change everything.

'That was exhilarating, wasn't it!' she exclaimed as the females formed a private circle.

'If you call getting hot, bothered and frustrated exhilarating!' said Carmel with a laugh as she pulled on a fresh pair of pants. 'It seemed to take about ten goes to do everything.'

Jack waited to one side until his charges were more decently clad and then came forward to address them.

'Well, I can see you have worked hard. Any problems?'

'Only working in a straightjacket,' replied Bud. The others nodded in accordance, Helen being the exception. Bud continued, 'It would be much easier with more help . . .'

'The Captain has spoken,' interrupted Jack. 'Even having Helen lurking about with the doors open is stretching things a bit. Anyway . . . how about coming back to some gravity for a bit and you can continue. I know it's a slow process, but that's the way it is.'

This time Bud interrupted. 'Oh! we don't really mind.'

'No, it's really exhilarating,' chimed in Stephanie.

'I was just thinking that if it's urgent to complete the job, more hands would speed it up,' concluded Bud.

Jack just nodded. He knew that Adam's directive had been a compromise between speed and safety, so he didn't really know how to respond to Bud's statement. They returned to a small common area near the main computer centre and relaxed with a drink each. Alan suddenly spoke. 'I don't suppose that anyone saw anything out there,' he stated almost apologetically.

'Just a few sirens, Ulysses,' replied Bud with a laugh.

'There were flashes directly in front of us when we pointed forwards,' said Carmel more soberly.

Helen nodded. 'Yes, when I wasn't looking back at you all, I noticed them when I looked forward.' Helen noticed Jack frown and continued, 'I didn't go out, boss, just had a peek over the edge!'

'No, that's all right, Helen,' said Jack, realising that

Helen had misinterpreted his expression.

'Did you see something else?' he asked Alan.

Everyone turned to Alan who took a minute to answer.

'Some flashes to the side of us . . .'

Stephanie felt herself shudder again. Helen noticed her reaction. 'Really, Alan! Look, you're giving poor Steph the heebie-jeebies!'

Jack, looking somewhat pensive, wondered whether the total void had caused Alan to hallucinate.

'It was when I turned my head in a certain direction,' stated Alan with more conviction, 'but it was difficult to keep in view.'

Everyone was too exhausted to pursue the matter any further, however, Jack ordered a two hour rest period and they all trooped off to their quarters.

Feeling refreshed and revitalised, they assembled once more. Jack had toyed with the idea of sending a different group, but Bud quickly pointed out that the first group had developed a certain degree of speed and efficiency and he prevailed upon Jack to allow them to continue.

Bud's thoughts proved correct as the original team worked much more efficiently on the second excursion. Most manoeuvres required two pairs of hands and Bud wished that he had a fifth team member, so that he could adopt a more supervisory role. He relied, however, on the interaction of voice commands and responses of his team, and they had it down to a fine art, resisting the temptation to indulge in small talk or expel unnecessary exclamations. There's nothing like practice, thought Bud, pleased with the ever increasing efficiency of his team, for whom he had a high admiration. The whole operation was approaching completion as Carmel manipulated a spar into position, Alan controlled the other end and lined it up, ready for her to secure. However, something appeared to distract him, causing him to turn suddenly and knock his end of the apparatus. Carmel was on the point of attaching her end when, in response to Alan's mishap, her end swung and struck her at waist level, crushing her jet packs and catapulting her away from the craft.

'Uh . . .' was Carmel's only immediate response before she had a chance to realise her predicament. However, Helen's voice quickly rang out, 'Bud! Carmel's been knocked somehow. Off to port a bit and directly above!'

Helen's concise directions enabled Bud to quickly orientate himself and search the void. To his horror and that of the others she seemed to be disappearing rapidly from view. Carmel didn't speak. To her horror she discovered the destroyed jet pack, crushed by the mishap. She grasped her line gun, mentally cursing the restriction of her gloves as she attempted to manipulate it in the correct direction. She seemed to be moving out of range rapidly. She took quick aim and fired. It would have been a perfect shot had it not skidded off the edge of the gantry that she had, moments before, been constructing.

Bud reacted quickly to the sudden crisis. Having orientated himself in Carmel's direction he activated his jets and set off apace. Even at maximum power it took some time to overhaul her. He was also conscious of the limited range of the jets, so once in range he took careful aim with the line gun and fired. A dull 'clunk' resounded in Carmel's helmet and she temporarily accelerated, then felt a pull as Bud hauled her to safety. The brief moment of terror over, she now suffered the indignity of being reeled in head first, not daring to alter her position through fear of breaking her tenuous lifeline. She also suffered the chilling sensation of staring directly into the void, but as she was towed back she had a sensation of intermittent streaks of light. The others, including Bud, came up beside her as she was reunited with the superstructure. No one had spoken lest they distract Bud from his task and in case he had any commands. Helen had activated a mobile unit, referred to by the techs as the 'tug', fearing that the rescue may have needed support.

'You OK?' said Bud, breaking the silence.

'Fine, thanks to you, Bud. I'm sorry, the spar just hit me and . . .'

'It was my fault,' interjected Alan. 'Something flashed in my face and I flinched and knocked the beam into Carmel.'

'No harm done,' said Bud, in turn interrupting Alan. 'We have to expect these mishaps. It's all part of the job.'

Bud's words had a distinctly calming effect on the group. Little did they know that his heart was fairly leaping out of his chest. He suppressed his excitement, however, for the sake of morale. He continued his calm approach to the situation by ordering everyone back to work. 'Very well. If you fall off a horse, best thing to do is to get right back on. That all right with you, Carmel?'

'Definitely,' came the reply, Carmel being inspired by Bud's trust.

'Just tie yourself on with one of the stray lines. That way, if you decide to go walkabout again, you'll take us all with you! We should be finished soon anyway.'

Finished they were in approximately twenty minutes. Bud piggy-backed Carmel back to the docking area where Helen eagerly awaited their arrival. Once inside, repressurisation began. A row of green lights signalled its completion as well as signifying to the group that they could safely disrobe. A communal sigh of relief could be heard as the suits were discarded; even Helen was red-faced on this occasion, the excitement of the rescue still foremost in her mind. Having stowed the exterior suits, they grabbed their clothes, worrying little about their appearance, and returned to 'civilisation', as Bud called it. Carmel gripped Bud's arm as he led them back. The realisation of her flirtation with danger was beginning to take effect. Once back in gravity, they flopped on the floor in a dishevelled heap, all semi-naked, with hair matted and comically pointing in all directions and clutching their overgarments.

'How about a wash and polish, then a bit of debriefing?' said Bud, hauling himself up.

A row of heads nodded in response and the group reassembled half an hour later. Alan recounted the event that had caused the distraction which had led to Carmel's unexpected propulsion into space. Carmel also related the flashing sensation that she had experienced on her undignified return journey.

'Anyone else see anything?' asked Bud, who had been far too preoccupied to bother with flashing lights.

'Yes . . .' said Stephanie.

They all turned to her. In appearance she had undergone an amazing transformation, now beautifully groomed, complete with make-up.

'A round bright object . . . just briefly, as Carmel was being pulled back.' She grinned as she spoke, recalling the undignified sight.

'Jack will be here in a minute,' said Bud, 'let's see what he makes of all this.'

Jack entered the room, as if by request, on the end of Bud's sentence.

'All done?' he said cheerily. I'm sorry I couldn't watch but the rest of us had to do your work whilst you were playing around out there, but I assumed that Helen would keep an eye on you and let me know if anything was amiss.'

Helen blushed. In amongst the drama, she hadn't thought of notifying Jack. Her expression and that on every other face transmitted the vibes to Jack that all had not been straightforward.

'Is there something I should know about?' he asked.

'Yes, chief,' replied Bud and he recounted the details of the mishap along with the accounts of the strange illuminations.

They watched as Jack momentarily contemplated his next remark.

'The cameras were on?' he asked in due course.

'Yes,' replied Helen, who had activated them as the group had left the docking area. The others heaved a sigh of relief. No one else, including Bud, had even given filming their task a thought.

'So which cameras were on?' asked Jack, turning to Helen.

'The wide angle from the dock, the tail and one directly beneath the workers.'

'Are you lot up to watching the movies, or do you want a rest?' continued Jack.

Everyone was much too excited to rest at that particular moment. Helen retrieved the films and the viewing commenced.

'Try the wide angle first,' suggested Jack.

The film began at the point Carmel was struck. It was halted and replayed, but nothing untoward was apparent; similarly nothing but blackness surrounded Carmel as she was hauled back.

'OK, let's try the one underneath,' said Jack.

This film provided a picture of the belly of the superstructure but little else.

'Take three?' said Helen, as she loaded the final film. Jack nodded.

The final film provided the best orientation of all, particularly of the accident. They gasped as the spar struck Carmel, this shot showing the event far more dramatically, including the splintering of her jet pack. At the same time, almost directly above her, where Alan was working, they clearly saw an intense dot like flash.

'That was it!' exclaimed Alan, 'I was afraid that I must have imagined it.'

Helen rewound the tape and paused the significant frames. There was no mistaking the intensity of the light source, but what did it represent they wondered? Helen advanced the film again, this time slowing down during Carmel's rescue. The picture was slightly obscured by the superstructure and Bud himself. Some flashes were seen, and then . . .

'Stephanie's round object!' exclaimed Bud.

The object only appeared on a few frames and disappeared. The group fell silent. Eventually Jack spoke.

'Well, I wonder what our clever scientists will make of that!'

Jack congratulated his team on a job well done, particularly in the light of the unexpected complications. All the more reason why I should have been supervising, he thought. He stood them down and advised them to rest until further notice; then, armed with the films of their adventures, he set off in the direction of the command centre. To his surprise, he found Yvonne instead of Adam.

'David finally prevailed upon Adam to rest,' explained Yvonne. 'I'm your temporary commander!' She made a mock curtsy as she spoke, much to Jack's amusement as he contrasted her personality to that of Adam's.

'How did you boffins make out with your new formulae?' asked Jack as he deposited the films on the console.

'We're getting there,' replied Yvonne, her eyes dropping to the films.

'Well, I've got some more food for thought,' stated Jack, placing his right hand on the three cassettes.

'Some films! Not more hanky panky, I hope, in our current situation . . .'

'Not exactly,' said Jack more sternly, 'the techs have completed the construction and assembly of the ion gun.'

'You don't waste any time. Well done. Are you going

to show me how they did it?'

'Sort of . . . you see there was a mishap . . .'

'A mishap! Anything serious?'

'All's well that ends well,' replied Jack. 'No, there was an accident but they handled the situation well.'

'Lucky you're telling me and not Adam; otherwise you would be receiving an earful of "I told you so".'

'It's probably best if I play the film and talk as I go,' said Jack, wishing to accomplish his mission. 'The tail camera captured it best, though you can look at the other films as well, but they don't show much.'

Jack advanced the film to the point of the accident. As it approached he said, 'You will see Alan, distracted, knock the spar into Carmel . . .'

Yvonne studied the screen closely, especially when Jack paused the frame with the intense light source. He then moved the film on. Yvonne gasped as the spar collided with Carmel, the shattering of the jet pack making it appear even more dramatic. She watched wide-eyed, as the rescue unfolded, like a child spellbound with an adventure film. As Carmel was towed in again Jack demonstrated the other light phenomenon. At the completion of the film Yvonne asked for it to be returned to the frames where the strange phenomena had occurred. She made a few sketches, then fanned her face with the notepad.

'I'm feeling hot!' she exclaimed, unzipping the front of her suit and fanning down onto her chest. 'This is very exciting, Jack!'

With that Yvonne rested back, arched her spine and ran her fingers through her hair. Jack said nothing; he knew that she would speak when ready. With her eyes pointed at the ceiling she flopped her wrist out languidly, offering her sketch for Jack's opinion.

'What do you think?' she asked, maintaining her upwards gaze.

Jack studied her artistry and said, 'A planetary system . . . at least . . . a solar system!'

Yvonne turned to face him, exposing her bare chest and with a broad smile said, 'Exactly!'

9

Adam flopped onto his bed, physically tired though mentally alert still, so he thought. How can I possibly sleep? he thought. His brain had no time to respond to the question; a deep coma was rapidly overtaking it. He awoke with a start approximately six hours later. He felt groggy and disorientated, in a much worse state than when he had embarked on the sleep which was supposed to refresh him. He groped for a cup of water to relieve his raging thirst and turned up the light slightly. He started as he suddenly noticed that he was not alone. In spite of his stirrings whoever it was continued to breathe heavily. Adam turned up the light a little more.

'Maria! What on Earth . . .' he hissed as he studied the semi-naked body sprawled next to him. He stood up, but much too quickly, the blood draining to his feet and making him dizzy. He lowered his head and repeated the manoeuvre, he really did feel wretched, not to mention confused. He rummaged for some clothes, only to find Maria's instead. Somehow, out of instinct, he pressed the intercom to the bridge. Yvonne's face appeared.

'Adam! Goodness you look a sight. Welcome back to the land of the living!'

'I've just woken up,' came Adam's croaky reply. 'Everything all right up there?'

'No problems at present, the techs have finished outside.

By the way, Adam, you have a nice body!'

Adam, suddenly aware of his nakedness, stuttered in reply. 'I . . . I . . . couldn't find my clothes . . . I woke up out of an incredibly deep sleep. That's good news about the exterior work . . . and by the way Maria's in my bed!'

Yvonne smiled at Adam's garbled statements. The revelation about Maria made her giggle. She composed herself and replied. 'Do you want me to give you some instructions on what to do?'

'It isn't what you think,' interrupted Adam. 'Never mind, I'll be with you shortly.'

Adam turned again to Maria. His conversation with Yvonne had not woken her. He rounded up his clothes, then dressed and stole away from his room and headed for the bridge. As he approached, Henny appeared with a plate of appetisers.

'These are for you . . . Yvonne ordered them.'

Adam felt a little better after his walk and the sight of Henny's handiwork caused him to feel better still.

'Come in and join us,' said Adam, ushering Henny in first. Henny appeared doubtful, but Adam insisted.

'It will be my pleasure,' he said, thinking that a conversation with Henny might be infinitely less stressful than those he was enduring with the scientists.

'This is your idea, I gather,' said Adam, waving in Henny's direction.

'I thought you might be a bit hungry,' replied Yvonne. 'Besides some are for me.'

Henny gazed around the command centre. Her visits to this part of the craft were rare; in fact Adam could not recall her being there at all previously. He put his thoughts into words.

'Have you been here before, Henny?'

'Only on orientation. Before we departed, it wasn't all lit up then.'

Adam and Yvonne munched on some sandwiches, whilst Henny's eyes continued to rove about the area. Adam eventually spoke again.

'How's the mood in your area, Henny? I mean the morale, given our circumstances . . .'

'He wants to know whether you are all scared witless like the rest of us,' Yvonne interjected.

Adam frowned at the un-commander-like statement, though the tone Yvonne had used suggested that she was anything but fearful.

'Very subtle,' said Adam, glaring at Yvonne.

'You have our complete confidence, Captain,' said Henny, collecting her thoughts. 'You too, Commander, we know how clever you are at working things out. After all, everything's working normally, isn't it?'

Henny's simple remark did more for Adam's confidence than a month of psychotherapy. He and Yvonne chatted with their guest for a short time; then Henny excused herself and left. Before either Adam or Yvonne could resume conversation, Maria appeared. The *femme fatale*, thought Yvonne, a smile breaking out across her face. Maria looked rather sheepish, though it was obvious that she had just woken up.

'Maria!' exclaimed Adam. 'A few minutes ago you were dead to the world.'

'Would you like me to leave?' asked Yvonne with a smirk.

'No, of course not,' retorted Adam. 'At least . . .'

'I'll explain,' interrupted Maria. 'I was feeling a bit down . . . lonely, or whatever, especially after all the scientific mumbo jumbo. I walked past your door, Adam, I just needed to be with a human being . . .'

'And you chose Adam?' laughed Yvonne. Maria just grinned, whilst Adam just sat with his eyes apparently out of focus.

'Well anyway,' said Maria, 'I went in. You were unconscious, Adam, I've never seen anyone in such a deep sleep, so I thought that you wouldn't mind if I just . . . I mean could be near you, so I took off my clothes and climbed in; I must have been alseep in seconds.'

'Yes I found the clothes all right . . . I nearly ended up wearing them,' remarked Adam.

'I'm sorry . . .' began Maria, but Yvonne promptly interjected. 'For goodness sake, don't apologise Maria, any man on board would relish your naked body next to him. Just because our illustrious captain missed his opportunity . . .'

'She wasn't completely naked,' interrupted Adam, though he recalled that Maria's only covering had been a flimsy T-shirt which barely reached to her waist. Yvonne would dearly have loved to provoke her two colleagues further, but duty suddenly rallied her thoughts.

'I'm sorry to break up the soap opera, you two, but there's some business which requires attention. Firstly, the techs have finished their work outside.'

That will take their mind off their personal relationships, she thought. Just in case it didn't, she added. 'They did have a mishap, though!' Yvonne paused as if to dramatise her statement. Her strategy proved successful as Adam blurted. 'What sort of mishap? Why wasn't I told?'

'They proved quite capable of handling the situation themselves. Do you really want to know every time someone burns the toast?'

'Not exactly a good analogy,' replied Adam, firmly. 'Very well . . . what happened?'

Yvonne knew that it was time to completely cease playing the joker; she gave an account of the events and showed the film. Adam and Maria watched intently.

'I'd like to get a first hand version from them,' said Adam, reaching for the intercom. Yvonne interrupted,

'Actually, Adam, they were pretty exhausted. Jack stood them down, and sent them to rest.'

Little did Yvonne know that at least two of the group, Carmel and Bud, were wide awake, the latter being rewarded by his rescued damsel in the nicest possible way. Fortunately, as a result of Yvonne's remark, they remained uninterrupted. Having regained Adam's attention, Yvonne continued, 'I'll explain my latest theories. Then we should be in a position to regain control.'

'Exactly how precarious is our situation then?' asked Adam.

'Well . . . I believe that what distracted the techs outside was a star system, at least its appearance as we whizzed past it in some point in space and time. Remember that we have postulated that we are moving in some relation to the axis along which the whole universe is moving.'

Maria frowned and said, 'It makes sense of course, but without any guidance, we could very well collide with something.'

'I thought of that,' replied Yvonne, 'I guess we are protected to a degree by the vastness of space itself, so the chances of us hitting something are slim.'

'But it's a concern, obviously,' said Adam. 'How do we work out where we are?'

'The only way would be to return to sub light speed and check,' said Yvonne. 'We can tell by the configuration of the known galaxy exactly where we are and when, in relation to current Earth time.'

'That will be interesting,' said Maria. 'We were pointed at Proxima Centauri, at least where it should be. When we return to our normal frame of reference, we should be able to calculate how far off course we are, so to speak, and determine the exact direction and speed of the universe itself. With that knowledge, it would become child's play to visit anywhere you liked!'

‘I know that this is very exciting and opens up lots of possibilities,’ said Adam, ‘but remember that this craft was not designed with such adventures in mind, so don’t go arranging any excursions to Andromeda!’

‘Don’t worry, Adam, I don’t think that our position will be necessarily that much different to what we expect. Basically, if we are flying in the direction of the universe or some vector to it, then we won’t be as close to Proxima as we should be; vice versa, if we are flying against its motion, we will be closer,’ said Yvonne.

The three colleagues sat and absorbed the ramifications of their discussion. They would repeat it again when Alex joined them later. The possibility of winding up close to another star system produced feelings of elation and apprehension. Adam, in particular, viewed the possibility with some trepidation. He called for a full report on their provisions. Also the return journey worried him. How much of the superacceleration had resulted from blind chance? Could they repeat it? Should they repeat it? If stranded in another system, would there be a suitable planet to replenish? He dismissed these thoughts and focused on the immediate plan to brake the DSP.

A feverish excitement gripped the crew as the objectives were promulgated. Some crew members were apprehensive, but all were optimistic and looked forward to the next phase of the adventure which had usurped the once mundane mission. Adam had asked Jack to study the possibility of landing on a distant planet or moon. Though only a faint possibility, Adam thought it necessary to anticipate. Jack mulled over the possibility with Bud.

‘It’s hard to plan when we have no idea what conditions we will be up against,’ said Jack. ‘I assume though that we would not approach anything with gravity greater than that on Earth.’

‘If it’s just a moon, it would be a piece of cake,’ replied

Bud.

'I know, but can you imagine the situation if we discover an Earth-like planet, and we are unable to visit it? We'd go crazy with frustration!'

One thing the designers of the DSP had blessed the craft with, was plenty of space. The rudiments of a landing craft were also provided; no one, it seems, really knew why. It just seemed logical that they should have one.

Helen, Yvonne and Carmel were engaged in a similar conversation as they established the internal connections and programming for the ion gun which the techs had assembled outside. They eventually took a break and began to fantasise about the future.

'I wonder if we'll find any nice Centaurian men . . .?' remarked Helen.

'Well . . . our part of the galaxy evolved about the same time and presumably in a similar fashion,' replied Yvonne, 'so there may be more similarities than we think.'

'Just as long as they're not hostile,' said Carmel. 'I must admit I'm a bit apprehensive.'

'When we get this contraption functioning, we can slow down and see where we are going,' said Yvonne, gesticulating towards a graphic representation of the newly constructed exterior gantry.

Carmel suddenly yawned. She looked tired and washed out.

'Too much bed and not enough sleep?' said Helen with a titter.

Carmel blushed and responded, sounding guilty. 'Boy nothing's private around here.'

The other two laughed. Yvonne soon added her own spice to the conversation by recounting the story of Adam, wakening and finding the naked and nubile Maria in his bed.

'She should be so lucky,' said Helen.

'I don't think she felt so lucky,' said Yvonne, 'it appears that she climbed out as innocent as she climbed in! Anyway, Helen, whilst we're on about true confessions, how's your love life?'

Now it was Helen's turn to blush as she faltered for an answer. Yvonne continued for her. 'I see,' said Yvonne, laughing, 'I'm getting the picture now . . . that walk in space seems to have turned you all into nymphomaniacs!'

Helen found her voice and replied, 'It was probably our ravenous naked bodies, when we peeled off our suits . . .'

'Or our beetroot faces and matted hair.' laughed Carmel.

'Actually, it was all in the line of duty,' continued Helen, 'Carmel was obliged to repay her rescuer . . . and I . . . I . . . well . . . absolved the guilt feelings of the individual who batted her into the never never.'

'Such devotion to duty,' said Yvonne. 'That does it . . . I'm coming on the next space walk if it's such an aphrodisiac!'

Helen laughed. 'You do all right, Yvonne . . . er . . . I seem to remember a certain person involved in the infamous nude frisbee match earlier in the trip. Don't tell me that you went quietly back to your own bed after that.'

'I went to my own bed . . . but I wasn't quiet!' came Yvonne's reply, following which she threw back her head and laughed wickedly.

'We're nothing but a pack of trollops,' gasped Helen amongst spasms of laughter.

The comedy was untimely interrupted by Jack, who appeared on the intercom. Three beaming faces greeted him at his end.

'How's it going down there?'

'We're well on the way Jack. We're just taking a break to . . . er . . . discuss a few things' . . .

A wry grin appeared on Jack's face. I can imagine, he thought to himself. Put a group of females together . . .

I'll bet the 'discussion' is about everything other than work.

Yvonne spoke again, having regained some decorum.

'If we can work around the clock, Jack, in shifts, everything should be on line in about forty eight hours.'

'Good work, girls, don't let me interfere with your . . . er . . . discussion, I just wanted to keep in touch.'

'I guess it's back to work,' said Yvonne, turning to her colleagues, 'though I haven't had such a good laugh for ages.'

'I'm glad our sex lives are such a source of amusement,' said Helen, rekindling the humour of their previous discussion.

'Just as long as they aren't a joke!' laughed Yvonne. 'That's enough. To work!'

10

Adam had his finger poised on the button . . . literally. He was about to take control of the DSP for the first time since they had been catapulted into their new dimension. With the moral support of his co-commanders, he mulled over their situation. Had his colleagues drawn the right conclusions and made the correct calculations? They seemed confident enough, yet they were confident before as well . . . and look what had happened! Yet perhaps he was taking his own responsibility far too seriously and not savouring the adventure itself. After all, what would ever have been discovered if explorers never took risks? That was the answer, he decided. In commanding the DSP, he had lost sight of the fact that, after all, they were on a voyage of exploration; otherwise they may as well be sailing a boat around a harbour, just to gain the experience of day to day duties.

Adam suddenly became aware that his colleagues all had their eyes fixed upon him, obviously awaiting his command. He refocused his thoughts and gave the order.

'Ten seconds . . . stand by.'

The countdown completed, reverse thrust was applied through the conventional engines in two second bursts, each five minutes apart. The commanders watched with fascination as their speed literally 'died' before their eyes.

As their speed decayed, however, warning lights began to appear and the crew became aware of a fine vibration throughout the craft. Adam shot a look at Alex and snapped, 'Should we continue?'

Alex's immediate response was a frown; only twenty seconds remained before the next burn was due.

'One more burn . . . then perhaps we should shut down.'

The vibration intensified during this final brief burst of retro thrust; Adam then cancelled the programme. Gradually the vibration faded and their speed levelled at twice light speed.

The anxiety level in the crew had steadily mounted in parallel with the intensity of the vibration, a similar wave of relief now ebbed as it subsided. Similarly most of the warnings disappeared.

'Any damage?' snapped Adam.

'Some on our new contraption,' replied Maria, 'otherwise nothing obvious.'

'At least we managed to get our speed down most of the way,' said Alex.

'What's our best course of action?' asked Adam.

'Use the ion gun . . . and decelerate more slowly, I suspect,' answered Alex.

'It sounds like it will need some repairs first,' said Adam, 'in the meantime we'll stand down.'

Adam immediately arranged a meeting with Jack.

'What do you make of the damage?' asked Adam.

'Probably a few loose nuts and bolts, so to speak,' replied Jack, 'but we need to look more closely of course . . . A fibre optic cable seems to have come adrift as well.'

'How long will it take to repair, do you think?'

'Probably a few hours. It's mainly inspection and adjustment. There shouldn't be any danger this time; they won't be waving any iron bars around and playing snooker with each other!'

Adam grinned at Jack's irrepressible humour. 'It'll take the brains a while to redo their calculations anyway, so there's probably no hurry,' he continued.

'I'll send four out . . . no need for any more than that,' concluded Jack, who then left to assemble his team. En route Maria suddenly approached him.

'Jack?'

Jack swung around. 'Maria . . . yes!'

'You'll be sending a team outside, won't you . . .?'

'Yes, I'm just about to organise . . .'

'I'd like to go along,' she interrupted.

Jack thought for a minute and shrugged. 'I don't see why not if you want to. Any particular reason?'

'Partly curiosity, I guess. But I would like to inspect any damage first hand. It might help us when we try the next manoeuvre.'

'Well, it's certainly all right with me,' said Jack. 'You'll check with Adam?'

'Of course.'

'I'll be down in our briefing area. Will you come down when you're ready?'

'I'll be back in a flash,' replied Maria, sounding excited. She swivelled and walked briskly back to confront Adam.

Having announced her intentions, Maria was subjected to a penetrating stare by Adam. She tried to allay what she thought may be his fears.

'I don't believe that there is any risk involved . . .'

'You can never say that for sure,' interrupted Adam, 'after all look what happened last time!'

'That was a much bigger operation. I just feel that one of us should see first hand . . .'

'And have a bit of an adventure?'

'Yes, that too . . . I'll admit it,' said Maria grinning. 'Look, I know that you are a bit reluctant about senior personnel going out there. That's why Jack delegates. Well,

. . . you can delegate to me. Apart from that certain circumstances dictate that the most senior ought to supervise and . . .'

'Don't worry, Maria, I won't play the heavy. As you know, you don't even need my permission to go. Besides . . . I do take your point.'

Maria wondered exactly which point Adam took, but she didn't pursue the matter, lest the debate be reactivated. Instead, in response to a sudden wave of physical attraction, she stepped forward, gave her captain a hug and left.

Adam called after her. 'Just be careful . . . I don't want to see you being hauled in like a harpooned whale!'

'Not me . . .' came Maria's response as she disappeared into the corridor.

Adam shook his head and muttered, 'The whole crew would end up wandering around out there, if I gave them half the chance!'

It would be an all female group that would exit the DSP, Helen in charge, with Carmel, Stephanie and Maria. The group assembled in the docking area, disrobed and clambered into the exterior suits. Maria slid her lithe body into the suit with a skill that the others admired. In spite of the suit's restrictions she would appear much less hampered than her colleagues. She relished the weightless environment and used her gymnastic training to good effect, enjoying the freedom which weightlessness provided. Once outside, Helen imposed strict silence upon the group, except for direct commands or responses.

Apart from providing an extra pair of hands when needed, Maria asked Helen for permission to inspect the superstructure. She noticed some small pits and fine radiating lines. She called Helen's attention and Carmel, being nearest, was dispatched to check the finding.

'What do you think?' asked Helen.

'It's not normal,' came the reply from Carmel.

'Check the whole length . . . Steph . . . come with me, we'll do this side,' ordered Helen.

The two pairs moved along their respective spars, then rendezvoused in a group at the base. Helen, having been nominally in charge, now deferred to Maria for her opinion.

'There's no doubt the superstructure has suffered some sort of fatigue, Maria, although it seems fairly superficial. What would you like us to do?'

'I suggest we complete the repairs, as planned, then I think it would be a good idea to make an inspection of the surface of the whole craft.'

'Very well. It shouldn't take us long to secure everything here. Carmel, you and I will check all the joints. Maria, can you assist Stephanie with the fibre optics?'

'Wilco . . .' replied Maria, hoping that she wasn't expected to know too much about the technical nature of her task. Stephanie, however, proved that she was an expert at the task and Maria proved an able assistant. Their job done, Helen contacted Jack.

'Jack, it's Helen, we need some advice . . .'

'Go ahead Helen. What have you found?'

'Some fine fatigue fractures on our new apparatus. I think that they are superficial, but Maria suggests that we check the skin of the craft itself.'

'That's a tall order, but I agree. This craft was not designed for vibration. I'll ask Adam to let the rest of us out, he shouldn't have any objection.'

Jack knew very well that Adam would not be pleased about his suggestion, but there was no question in Jack's mind about improved efficiency if he used all his personnel.

Predictably, Adam began to pace up and down on hearing Jack's recommendation.

'I agree, Jack, that it's necessary. It just goes against

the grain authorising the whole technical complement . . .'

'It's the best way, Cap. Really we are designed to work as a team. This itty bitty approach just isn't appropriate. I took your point before, during the construction, but this is an inspection, it's . . .'

'Different,' said Adam, completing the sentence. 'Very well, Jack, you've convinced me!'

'I'll leave Bud inside,' said Jack, 'I really think that I should go on this one.'

Adam nodded, pleased that he had one member of the technical team left aboard. Jack then hastened to the docking area. It wasn't long before he, Alan and Bernard were outside and mingling with their female colleagues.

'Coming out to even up the sex ratio?' quipped Maria, before the command structure became reformalised. Jack, who always enjoyed a bit of friendly banter responded, 'OK my bevy of beauties, the captain's pacing up and down inside like a caged lion, so any trouble and I'll get a net and haul you in like a sack of tuna.'

'No sexist language, Jack,' came the reply from Maria, 'remember you guys are outnumbered.'

'I think we're pretty harmless in these suits,' concluded Jack.

With that remark, the frivolity ceased and the group fanned into a long horizontal line and advanced from the rear of the DSP. The inspection tour exhilarated Maria, after being cooped up inside for so long, especially as her duties dictated that she spend most of her time in the gravity areas. Not that the craft was particularly cramped, but to actually view their entire cocoon from the outside caused her to wonder at their whole situation; it also gave her an exhilarating sense of freedom. She occasionally glanced across at her colleagues, these unassuming Jacks and Jills of all trades were the lifeblood of the whole mission, she thought. She felt a sense of pride that she had inadvertently become a part of their activities.

She was careful not to allow her thoughts to distract her attention from the strip of the DSP to which she had been allotted. The external lighting gave the craft a surrealistic appearance and she noted that the beams of light arced slightly as they ran along the surface. She wondered about the scientific explanation for this. Otherwise, away from the craft, it was total blackness, except for her colleagues who were lit up like actors suspended in midair; like characters in a children's pantomime on wires, thought Maria.

As they came to the rotating gravitational area, Jack led his brood well away from the craft and instructed them to remain in a group, whilst he and Helen approached the moving target and joined its motion. When they rejoined the group, Jack held a mini-conference.

'Anything to report?'

They all answered, 'No', in a predetermined order. They then headed down the front of the craft and once again paused before commencing the return journey along the belly. During this space walk, Adam became a direct spectator via the external cameras, plus one that Jack had mounted on his suit to provide close up viewing of any unusual discoveries. Now, as the group started towards the rear, Maria said, 'I've found something Jack!'

'All halt,' ordered Jack at once, 'keep your positions.'

He moved across and joined Maria, focusing on the craft beneath her. His eyes widened at the sight of a multitude of fissures in the surface of the craft. He looked across at the others. 'Have a good look, everyone . . .'

'I can see some very fine lines . . . like crazy paving . . .' came Stephanie's voice as she recalled the appearance of her grandmother's pathway.

Jack contacted Adam. 'Adam, we've found some fissuring . . . it seems pretty superficial. Can you see it?

. . . I'll point the camera at it.'

Adam studied the picture intently.

'Is Bud with you Adam?' asked Jack.

'Yes, Jack.'

'Can you ask him to activate the nearest external oxygen port? We'll probably need some extra time out here.'

Bud, who was sitting next to Adam, nodded. 'I can do it from here, Cap . . .'

'Bud's activating it now, Jack,' relayed Adam.

'Right, I'll sign off from you, Cap . . .' said Jack. He then directed his group once more. 'Who can see the oxygen port?'

'It's right under me,' came the reply from Carmel.

'Very well. Best if you girls start first. You should be the lowest. You start Carmel.'

Adam and Bud watched as Carmel began to attach to the port. Having done so, the recharge only took a matter of seconds. Having completed the task, she leant forward in order to disengage. Then, to Adam and Bud's horror, she was catapulted violently off the surface by a huge blast from the port. Those on the outside were even more horror-struck as a large gash opened and a blast of ''gasicles'' sprayed them as they moved up to take their turn after Carmel.

Maria was immediately next to Carmel, the latter being flung against her with incredible force. Almost instinctively Maria arched, as much as the restrictive suit would allow, and grabbed wildly as Carmel ricocheted away. The collision had transferred some of Carmel's momentum and Maria, managing to grasp Carmel by the leg, re-equalised it to some degree, but they both spun uncontrollably away from the craft.

In spite of the blast, the collision with Maria and the violent spinning motion, and having Maria flailing off the end of one leg, Carmel had drawn her line gun and, when oriented towards the craft, which was rapidly disappearing, she aimed and fired. It was a brilliant shot . . . given the circumstances. She made a direct hit near the ruptured oxygen port which, however, had been replaced by a huge frozen gas ball. The end of the line bit, momentarily, then broke away with a large chunk of ice attached. The temporary tug cancelled the spinning motion but did little to prevent their rapid propulsion into space. Maria fired her line, once oriented, but too late. Other lines crisscrossed the void but the target proved too difficult to hit.

Carmel hauled Maria up to eye level, as if for reassurance, then barked, 'Line up your jet with mine and fire together. Three . . . two . . . one . . .'

Maria obeyed the command without question. There was no doubt in her mind that the level-headed Carmel should call the tune. The jets slowed their outward motion, but the initial blast had been powerful indeed and the jets, even in combination, could not reverse the direction of their motion. Maria gulped as she watched the craft diminish in size. The other members of the group had been scattered by the event, but now some had instinctively gone after the stricken pair. Jack had been temporarily unsighted by icicles. He now tried to restore order.

'Come back! Helen, Bernard, you'll never catch them! We need the tug . . .'

'I'm on my way . . .' came a voice in Jack's helmet. As it was female, he concluded that it must belong to Stephanie, who was the only one that he couldn't see. In fact Stephanie had summed up the gravity of the situation within seconds and had quickly realised that the tug was the only hope of rescuing her colleagues.

'Stephanie, where are you?' screamed Jack.

'Just entering the dock, Jack!' she replied to his amazement. He turned his attention to the victims and tried to sound reassuring. 'Carmel . . . Maria . . . hang on, we'll get you. Keep those jets oriented . . .'

Oriented the jets were. They produced strange oscillating forces to which Maria's body responded instinctively. Although diminutive, her gymnastic muscles were powerful and she held herself and Carmel in position. Carmel clung with one arm to her bamboo-like colleague.

The speed with which Stephanie had returned to the docking area was truly amazing. She had shaved minutes of the journey by risking a passage through the giant rotating gravity areas of the craft. The speed at which these giant bulges moved was considerable and required perfect judgement and precision in timing to avoid being kicked into space as well. However, Stephanie was a person with a determination to be reckoned with, and she had no intention of becoming the victim of another mishap. Of course her colleagues were still recovering from the accident as she weaved her dangerous path. Only Adam and Bud could see what she did and sat helpless and awestruck as the drama unfolded.

Maria broke silence. In a shaky voice she addressed Carmel. 'Looks like you get rescued again . . .'

'We're a long way from being rescued,' replied Carmel firmly. The DSP had become no more than a blob. The two stranded colleagues could not see the tug burst to life and pull their would-be rescuer into the void.

'I'm under way,' came Stephanie's voice. Her heart pounded. Why me? she thought. She scanned for her friends, eventually finding a dot in the matt black background. The rest of the group were helpless and began to drift back to the dock, taking the long way around, rather than Stephanie's more dangerous route. Jack was conscious of the fact that his most junior person held the fate of Maria and Carmel in her hands. He resisted the temptation to bark orders at her, particularly as she appeared to have the situation under control. Stephanie gripped the tug with such force that she thought that she would crush the handles; not that her gloves allowed that much flexibility. She had the power on maximum, which had the effect of pulling her suit forwards with a crushing force on a very sensitive area.

'Oooh . . . my fanny's being cut in half,' she thought she said aloud, although she couldn't be sure.

Jack's voice interrupted her thoughts. 'You're doing fine, Steph . . . like a pro . . .'

'I'm a bit freaked out, Jack . . .' she replied.

Jack recognised the pain in her response and made an instant diagnosis. 'Slacken off the acceleration every so often. It stops you from being pulled into the suit and helps you steer more easily.'

The voice of experience, thought Stephanie, as she imagined what dreadful injuries would befall a male in the same situation. Jack spoke again.

There's a safety strap on the body of the tug, did you connect it?'

'No.'

'Very well, do it now, so you don't become separated . . . especially when you reach the others.'

'Done.'

'There's a circle on the viewer. If you're using maximum power . . . when the subject fills it . . . ease off the power.'

'They're still just a dot and still moving away.'

'You'll overhaul them eventually, don't worry. There's plenty of fuel in the tug. It's just a matter of time . . .'

The 'time' seemed like an eternity to Stephanie; her pupils were dilated to maximum. The only recording her eyes made was the dot which represented her target.

Alex and Yvonne had joined Adam and Bud in the command centre.

'Can we manouevre the DSP any closer?' asked Adam.

Alex shook his head. 'No. I know they seem a long way

away but we'd just run them down.'

Yvonne and Bud both agreed.

'What about the rupture?' said Adam, suddenly turning his thoughts to the cause of the accident.

'It will seal with frozen gas,' replied Bud, 'but I had better go down and turn off a few taps and isolate the area.'

Adam nodded in response and Bud left.

David had also joined Adam and his colleagues on the bridge.

'How far are they away now?' he asked.'

'About three kilometres,' replied Adam.

'What's Stephanie like?' continued David.

'She's the youngest and least experienced,' replied Adam bluntly.

'Let's hope she's a fast learner,' thought David, but he remained silent.

Unbeknown to most, alarms began ringing almost simultaneously in the helmets of Helen, Maria and Stephanie. 'Damn, the oxygen,' muttered Stephanie.

'Jack, my oxygen's down to ten minutes, which means . . .' said Helen.

Jack interrupted. 'Steph . . . Maria . . .'

'Yes Jack, the bells are ringing,' replied Stephanie, nervously.

Maria responded immediately. 'I can share with Carmel . . . and we'll top you up when you get here, Steph!'

His heart having missed a beat or two, Jack sighed with relief as he realised that the cause of the whole predicament, namely Carmel's oxygen replenishment, would save the day . . providing nothing else went wrong. But something did go wrong . . . horribly wrong! The oxygen alarm worked on a time basis. It was a rough guide only, no one assuming that the level would be allowed to fall so low before replenishment. It also worked on an average consumption basis, but Stephanie's consumption had been far from average. Apart from the initial physical manouevering, her concentration and anxiety had combined to burn the precious gas at a furious rate. Her head began to pound and the continuous alarm gnawed at her sanity.

She spoke, mainly to keep her senses. 'I have a problem . . . stand by . . .'

Carmel and Maria straightened in response to the signal from Stephanie. They had completed the oxygen-sharing manouevre and could see the tug approaching quite clearly. No one dared speak. To Carmel's horror, she could see the tug's course start to waver.

'I . . . I . . . can't . . . I . . . can't hold it . . . I . . . Carmel . . . I'm pulling off course . . .'

Then suddenly Stephanie managed one last lucid statement. 'I'll line up and detach . . .'

Carmel screamed in response, 'Don't you dare . . . you little brat . . . no . . . I'll smack your bum if you do . . . Stephanie . . . stay awake . . .'

There would be no reply as Stephanie's lifeless body drifted clear of the tug, which now continued its journey unmanned.

'It's going to miss us . . .' uttered Carmel as she watched the trajectory of the tug arc to one side. Maria suddenly flexed her hips and placing her feet against Carmel, she kicked away, propelling Carmel away in the opposite direction. At full extension Maria managed to just reach and tip the nose of the tug. The machine still travelled at considerable speed and in rotating sharply in Maria's direction, rammed hard against her glass face plate, smashing it.

Carmel had managed to re-orientate herself, though as a result of Maria using her as a launch pad, she had moved a considerable distance away and was still travelling.

Although Carmel did not see the collision, she saw the

effect. A cloud of frozen gas erupted about Maria's head. She also heard Maria's choking scream as her suit depressurised and the deathly cold struck her face. Those back on the DSP listened in blind horror as the rescue mission plunged into utter chaos. They had little visual contact, the drama being barely in range of the cameras. No one dared speak, almost as if they were in fear of interrupting the participants, of which there now only appeared one . . . Carmel, and what chance did she have?

Expecting to die within seconds, Maria spoke in a rasping screech. 'Carmel . . . my face plate . . . it's broken, I'm blind . . . my face . . . it's on fire.'

Carmel quickly realised that the fact that Maria was able to speak, could only mean one thing.

'Maria, the glass will seal. It's designed to. You're OK. Just don't let go of the tug. You'll have ice all over the face plate. That's why you can't see. Just don't let go!'

Maria had no intention of letting go. She clung to the shaft of the tug like grim death. Carmel was shaking. Furthermore, the distance between her and Maria was increasing at an alarming rate.

Maria suddenly uttered some reassuring words. 'I can just see out the sides of my mask . . . just.'

'Work your way along to the back. Then grab the bar with one hand. Don't let go with that hand . . . no matter what . . . Use the other hand for any manouevres. Do you know how to operate the tug?'

Any training that Maria might have had evaporated in the light of current events. 'I . . . I'm . . .'

'That's OK,' interrupted Carmel, correctly diagnosing Maria's dilemma. 'Just listen carefully. There's a joystick on the very top of the control panel. Don't touch anything else, just follow my instructions. Ready?'

'Ready!'

Carmel snapped instructions staccato style at Maria.

Eventually the tug loomed before her. She dared not risk trying to instruct Maria to attempt to slow it, lest she make a mistake. She knew that she only had one chance at rescue. This chance came quickly. She yelled at Maria just before the tug struck.

'Hold on . . . both hands . . . ugh!'

The force of the impact was transmitted dramatically through Carmel's suit. Once recovered, she quicky wormed her way along to the driver's end and secured Maria, then herself. She then cast her eyes about for Stephanie. She had lost her . . .

'Jack, anyone on board. Can you see Steph? Where is she . . . where . . .?'

Adam recognised the hysteria developing in Carmel's voice and immediately took charge.

'Carmel, this is Adam. We have Stephanie on the scanner. In relation to your nose, she's almost directly behind you, slightly to starboard and below.

Carmel quickly computed Adam's directions and swung the machine about. 'I've got her in sight. Stand by . . .'

Adam watched the screen of the scanner, occasionally flicking his eyes to the direct picture, which revealed little. He watched the two dots on the scanner come together. As they did so Carmel spoke, her voice starting to break up again.

'We have her. We have her . . .'

'Fine,' replied Adam calmly, his voice belying his inner emotions.

Carmel shook as she attempted to join the oxygen port onto the flaccid Stephanie, craning to see the face of her colleague but Stephanie's face was slumped forward. The task completed, Carmel spoke in a choking voice. 'She's not responding . . .'

'Bring her in Carmel,' came Adam's sober voice once more.

Carmel jabbed at the throttle. Unprepared, Maria suffered a painful collision with the crutch of her suit.

'Sorry, Maria,' said Carmel, realising what she had done. She also became aware of the pressure in an identical part of her own anatomy, but she cared little as she towed her colleagues back to the DSP.

Preparations for the arrival of the stricken group had preceded apace. The medical contingent of David, Anna, Loretta and Kate, floated outside the dock amidst a myriad of equipment.

'How long since we lost contact with Stephanie?' asked Loretta grimly.

'Believe it or not, less than five minutes. Yet it seems like an eternity,' replied David.

Loretta shivered in response to the word 'eternity'. Her senses sharpened as she mentally prepared herself for the task ahead.

In another section of the craft Yvonne all but choked as she recalled an earlier conversation with Maria in which they had experienced a vivid premonition of the fate which had befallen Stephanie. Meanwhile Carmel's return journey took considerably less time than Stephanie's outward sojourn, Stephanie having been hampered by the difficulty of keeping such a small target in view, and consequently unable to use full power all of the time. Carmel had no such restriction. In spite of the extra load the DSP loomed like a large whale and for most of the trip she continually accelerated. She would worry about braking when she got there.

Few words were spoken on that short journey back to safety. However, as the tug approached, Carmel spoke at last. 'I'll be detaching the other two. Get ready to catch.'

Those standing by in the airless dock weren't immediately certain of Carmel's intentions, but they had been concerned at how she would brake the tug, having driven it up to what seemed like an excessive speed. However, the resourceful young technician put the wide open dock carefully in her sights, then detached her colleagues. As she did so she sharply altered the direction of thrust. Maria and Stephanie sailed forward, continuing their original line of motion straight through the open doors of the dock, whilst Carmel, plus machine, arced away to the side. Carmel's calculations left little room for error as she all but skated across the surface of the DSP while fighting to bring the speeding craft to a halt.

Reacting quickly to the two figures who came sailing through the doors, those inside deftly spun and pushed their colleagues, quickly dissipating their momentum. Having avoided smashing herself and her machine to pieces, Carmel spoke breathlessly.

'Close up. I'll wait out here, just help Steph. Please . . .' She paused, then added, 'and Maria.' She suddenly realised that Maria had not spoken on the return journey.

The doors of the dock closed and the area rapidly repressurised. The medical team stormed inside as the two casualties were hauled from their suits. Helen, who assisted with Maria, gasped at the sight before her. Maria had a huge welt diagonally across her face. This in turn led into a laceration which extended from the angle of her left eyebrow into her scalp. The top of her head was a mass of matted hair and blood.

Mercifully, she spoke. 'I'm all right . . . help Stephanie!' she gasped. But Maria looked anything but all right. When completely free, it became apparent that more blood had seeped down her body, completely soaking the cotton liner that she wore.

Anna appeared at her side. 'Come with me,' she ordered and quickly led her out of the chamber in the direction of the clinical area. Meanwhile the lifeless Stephanie had been flung against a wall and pinned. A pair of scissors wielded by Loretta split the material covering her chest to which electrodes were instantly applied by David. Kate simultaneously had inserted an intravenous line on what she could see of an arm. As Kate raised her head after connecting her line, she caught sight of Stephanie's exposed breasts and momentarily shot a look at Loretta, whose eyes seemed to answer the question which Kate's expression posed. Both their heads turned quickly to the cardiac monitor. David in turn was already pumping oxygen into Stephanie's lungs.

'A heart beat . . . thank God . . . Although it looks bloody terrible . . .' ejaculated Loretta.

'It's a ventricular tachycardia. Shock her!' snapped David.

'Stand clear!' ordered Kate, as she applied the paddles. Stephanie's body convulsed violently in the weightless environment, causing Loretta to cry out, 'Christ almighty, I hope she hasn't broken anything!'

'Sinus rhythm . . .' David interjected, observing the successful result of the brutal electrocution.

'Is she breathing?' asked Kate.

David stopped pumping and the three transfixed their eyes on the bag which David allowed to sit loosely in the palm of his hand. It rippled slightly.

'Shallow . . .' said David and immediately resumed his pumping. 'Let's connect her up and move . . .' he continued and immediately attached Stephanie's airway to a respirator.

The medicos had been oblivious to the other personnel still in the chamber. The latter had marvelled at the speed and efficiency with which David, Loretta and Kate had worked to restore life to their colleague. Adam had observed the scene from the command centre, not interrupting lest he distract those on the spot. He waited until the medical team, with Stephanie in tow, had cleared the area, before taking charge again.

'Jack, get ready for Carmel to enter. Carmel, stand by. Are you ready?'

'Ready,' came Carmel's reply as she hovered immediately outside. A short time later she entered the deserted dock, dumping the tug. She then waited for the area to repressurise, a procedure which seemed to take forever. Finally a row of green lights appeared and simultaneously Helen burst into the chamber. She had Carmel desuited in what appeared like seconds.

Carmel coughed out just one word. 'Stephanie . . .'

'She's alive. They're on their way to the clinincal area. She's unconscious, though. They had to shock her.'

Carmel looked totally distraught and continually shook her head. Eventually she managed to speak. Helen noticed tears welling in her friend's eyes.

'That means her heart had stopped . . .'

'No, I don't think so. She had an abnormal beat or something. They shocked her to correct it.'

'Did it work?'

'Instantly!' replied Helen forcibly.

'Where are the others?' asked Carmel, suddenly realising that the place was deserted, apart from equipment and clothing floating everywhere. It made the place look very untidy.

Everyone's gone off to check on the oxygen port that exploded,' replied Helen. 'Come and get cleaned up, Carmel.'

Helen placed her arm around her exhausted friend and gripped her tightly.

The transfer from weightless to gravitational areas normally posed no difficulty, but the medical team found that it took some skill to propel Stephanie and her attached equipment through the window, so to speak. However, they executed the task with the same skill at which they had handled the resuscitation and a short time later entered the rarely used clinincal area of the craft.

As David, Loretta and Kate delivered their charge, they noticed that Anna had not been idle. She had Maria propped bolt upright. Her clothes were cut away and a splotch of brown antisceptic was smeared over her chest. There had been no time to clean away any of the blood and poor Maria presented a gruesome picture as she gasped desperately behind an oxygen mask.

'She's blown a pneumothorax. It must have happened when her suit repressurised suddenly, and it's getting worse . . .' said Anna sounding quite desperate herself.

'I'll help,' said Kate, immediately taking the initiative and dashing to Anna's side. 'Doesn't everything happen at once in this game.'

As David and Loretta installed Stephanie, Anna grasped a brutal looking, sharp metal, trochar and plunged it into Maria's delicate chest above her right breast. A hiss of air was immediately expelled, accompanied by a stifled cry of agony from the unfortunate Maria.

'Sorry, honey!' exclaimed Anna as she quickly threaded a tube and withdrew the hollow metal weapon which had savaged Maria's sylph-like body. Stitches were then inserted to maintain the position of the tube, whilst Kate connected the other end to an underwater seal.

'You'll feel better in a minute,' said Anna as she completed her stitching. Maria did feel better. She promptly fainted!

'Can we bring her down a bit?' asked Kate. 'She's lost a fair amount of blood . . .'

Anna and Kate both surveyed Maria's blood-smeared body and that which stained the remains of her clothing.

'OK but not too far. And we'll speed up that IV. Can you check her blood group?'

Kate nodded in response to the multiple requests and

complied with each one in turn. Thirty minutes later, the now dishevelled medical team stopped for the first time in ages, it seemed, to draw breath. Maria had swum back to consciousness, mainly in response to the stimulus of severe pain. She had been immediately dispatched back into semi-coma by a large dose of pain killer and sedation.

The restorers of life stood in an irregular line, their eyes moved back and forth between the victims of the mishap.

'I guess they're stable,' murmured David.

The others nodded.

'We'd better go and see the chief,' continued David, turning to Anna as he spoke. 'Are you girls happy to hold the fort?'

Loretta and Kate both nodded again. Some time later, after washing caked blood from Maria and cleaning away the rubble from the earlier procedures, the two nurses sat between their two patients and chatted in loud whispers as they tried to overcome the beeping of monitors, clicking of intravenous pumps and the whoosh of Stephanie's respirator.

'I didn't expect I'd be doing anything like this', said Loretta with a slight shake of the head. Kate nodded. Her mind was occupied with something else.

'How old do you reckon Stephanie is?'

'You noticed,' replied Loretta, 'I thought you did. It's pretty obvious. Those aren't the breasts of a mature woman. I also found she was padded when I cut away her clothes. What do you think?'

'Fourteen. Sixteen at the most,' whispered Kate.

They both turned to gaze at the inanimate young female next to them. They stared inquisitively at her face, the mouth distorted by the laryngeal tube.

'She looks much younger than she usually does,' continued Kate. 'But how . . . I mean how did she get selected? She obviously normally does herself up to look older.'

'However she did . . . or whatever else . . . she's saved two lives . . . and was prepared to sacrifice her own in the process . . .'

David and Anna arrived in the command centre to find Adam and Yvonne hungry for news.

'We didn't want to interrupt you,' began Adam.

'I know. Thanks, Adam. We appreciate it, but we knew that you would want to know. So we came as soon as we thought they were stable. We had some unexpected problems with Maria as well. She collapsed a lung, but she's OK now.'

Adam was momentarily taken aback by this unexpected news. 'And Stephanie?'

David sighed before he attempted to reply. Eventually he formulated his answer. 'There's no doubt that she suffered lack of oxygen for a significant period, though it was shorter than I would have originally estimated. She responded quickly to resuscitation . . . but I'm afraid . . . in cases like this . . . only time will tell.'

Adam shot a look at Anna, as if to immediately gain an instant second opinion. She responded to his inquiring expression. 'I agree with David. She has got youth on her side, of course.'

Adam nodded. He was aware that Stephanie was one of the younger members of the crew . . . not that anyone was particularly old.

'You'll keep me informed?' said Adam.

'Of course,' replied David.

With that David and Anna left and rejoined their nursing colleagues. Anna admired the transformation that had taken place in their absence.

'You've turned a bomb site into a palace,' she exclaimed. 'I'm sorry we ran off and left you to clean up the mess!'

'Typical doctors,' replied Kate laconically. 'We're used

to it!'

The group managed an abbreviated laugh before they returned to the business at hand.

'Stephanie's vital signs are good,' stated Loretta, 'and her pupils are reacting,' she added triumphantly.

'Maria's stable as well,' said Kate. 'She gets a bit restless from time to time, otherwise she's fine . . . except she looks horrible. I've been putting ice packs on that horrible bruise on her face.'

They stood in silence for a moment before Loretta spoke again. 'We were wondering about Stephanie's age . . .'

Anna appeared puzzled by the remark, but David said, 'I know what you mean . . .'

'What do you mean?' asked Anna.

'Take a close look at her Anna,' said Loretta.

Anna studied the dormant figure closely. Loretta pulled back the sheet covering Stephanie's upper body. Anna then concentrated on her face again. Loretta voiced the communal thoughts.

'Fourteen . . . sixteen at the most?'

'But it's impossible,' replied Anna, 'the minimum age for this mission was twenty-three. How . . .?'

'We may never know "how" if she doesn't wake up,' interjected David.

'Do we tell anyone?' asked Kate.

'I don't believe that there is any point at the moment,' continued David. 'Keep your ears open, though . . . I'd be willing to bet that someone else on board knows the story!'

11

'How bad is the damage, Jack? Are we about to open up like a sardine can?'

Jack's weary face managed half a smile in response to Adam's question, before he answered. 'I think not, Cap. You can forget about that oxygen port, of course. It sealed up straight away and we've isolated it as well. I suspect that we probably decelerated much too quickly, but we had no way of knowing that it would do any harm.'

'It's certainly hard to play safe when we don't know the rules,' said Adam ruefully. 'We have some good news, though. Maria's much better and Stephanie is showing definite signs of recovery, though they keep saying it's early days.'

'I feel somehow responsible,' said Jack, shaking his head.

'Don't,' replied Adam abruptly. 'I've been feeling just as guilty. It was just an incredible combination of circumstances. It was even more remarkable the way that the girls combined to get themselves out of it. We could have quite easily lost all of them.'

'But we learn from our mistakes,' continued Jack. 'There will certainly be some modifications to our safety procedures.'

'True,' said Adam, 'nothing teaches better than trial and error.'

His conference with Jack completed, Adam decided to

visit the clinical area. He found Loretta on duty alone. Maria was alseep. Stephanie still lay motionless, apart from a rhythmical jerking in response to the respirator. Loretta rose as Adam entered. Her steel-like eyes met his. Cool efficiency, combined with a kind mouth, thought Adam. The perfect nurse.

'This is a privilege!' whispered Loretta, extending her hand.

Adam gripped her hand rather than shaking it; a warmth seemed to flow from it. Adam gazed at Stephanie. Loretta wondered what his thoughts were.

'Dollar for your thoughts, Captain.'

'I must be getting old. She looks so young.'

Younger than you think! thought Loretta but she said nothing.

'What do you think her chances are?' asked Adam. 'She still needs the respirator . . .'

'Not really,' replied Loretta. 'In fact she'll be gradually coming off it soon. It's been left on to maximise her oxygen intake.'

Kate appeared at that moment and she also greeted Adam warmly, whereupon he praised both of them.

'You're doing an excellent job. I've certainly no fears of falling sick on this ship.'

'No one ever falls sick on this ship,' laughed Kate, 'you're all too damned fit and the food's so healthy . . .'

'Well, that's the way the mission was planned,' replied Adam. 'It's nice to see that aspect of it is working out OK.'

'The rest of it will work out as well,' said Loretta, feeling that her captain could probably do with a dose of reassurance.

Kate also added her bit. 'We're all a pack of mad adventurers, Captain. We have complete faith in you, though we can do without the spectacular accidents.'

'We'll do our best to avoid them,' replied Adam. 'This

one was a bit freakish, though.'

'I think Carmel's driving on the way back was freakish,' said Loretta. 'The time she saved almost certainly made the difference between life and death for both Stephanie and Maria.'

Adam nodded. 'We estimate that she cut up to ten minutes off that journey. Assuming it would have been conducted in the usual manner, she came within millimetres of crashing and killing herself. In fact it's ironic. Stephanie was willing to sacrifice her life on the way out for Carmel and Maria, and Carmel hers on the way back for Stephanie and Maria.'

'Have you spoken to Carmel?' asked Kate.

'No,' replied Adam, sounding guilty. 'Have you seen her?'

'Not seen. But she enquires constantly. David and Anna have steadfastly refused visitors . . . except for you of course.'

Adam thanked the nurses for their time and was soon back on the bridge, in conference with his co-commanders.

'I wonder if we can have a space walk without an accident!' exclaimed Adam.

'Well, we need one more to be completely sure that the inspection is complete,' stated Alex firmly.

'Very well,' said Adam bluntly. 'Two only . . . and two standing by in the dock, with the tug ready to go.'

Within minutes Bud and Alan were preparing to exit the craft whilst Helen and Bernard made ready the tug. Maria's bloodstained suit and splintered face plate still hung as grim reminders of what could go wrong. However, this time all went exactly to plan and Bud and Alan returned. They reported no further signs of damage and confirmed that the rupture had completely sealed.

Whilst her colleagues completed the task in which Stephanie was originally involved, she maintained her steady improvement. Her laryngeal tube had been removed and she breathed spontaneously. She also moved all of her limbs, albeit in a restless fashion, but enough to excite her medical attendants. Later they would have the satisfaction of seeing and hearing her respond to the sound of her name, even though it only consisted of a murmur. Loretta and Kate had settled into a routine of shifts, though sometimes they overlapped or were both relieved by David or Anna. It would be Loretta who would experience the spectacular turning point of Stephanie's recovery.

It would occur as Loretta was attending to Maria. The latter had been kept sedated most of the time, especially as she experienced considerable pain still from her facial injuries. As if receiving a telepathic message, Loretta looked across at Stephanie and to her amazement she noticed that her eyes were wide open and staring straight ahead. The lights were turned down quite low and Stephanie appeared not to see Loretta until she was almost upon her. Stephanie appeared startled as Loretta's presence registered.

'Gran . . .' uttered Stephanie, squinting in the gloom.

'It's Loretta. Steph, you're in the clinic.'

'I'm where?' replied Stephanie, sitting upright. At the same time she caught sight of the intravenous line in her arm and studied it intently.

'You had a nasty accident, honey . . .'

'I don't know what you mean,' interrupted Stephanie.

'You . . .'

'Who is that?' said Stephanie, suddenly catching sight of Maria. 'Is it Carmel?' she continued, once again choking off any reply from Loretta.

'No . . . it's Maria, she . . .'

'Where's Carmel?'

'She's fine . . . fit as a fiddle.'

Loretta decided that it was time to take command of the situation. She smiled reassuringly at Stephanie and gently eased her back into a resting position.

'You've nothing to worry about, Steph . . . just rest . . .'

Stephanie promptly obliged and seemed to fall asleep as suddenly as she has awakened. The slumber was short-lived however and Stephanie spoke again.

'Carmel . . . Carmel . . .'

Loretta moved to reassure her, but to no avail. She quickly raised David on the intercom and after acquainting him with the situation he suggested that Carmel visit. She materialised in what appeared like seconds. She stopped momentarily as she entered the clinic. In doing so Stephanie caught sight of her and pleaded. 'Carmel. Something's happened . . .'

Carmel rushed forward, stopped abruptly just out of reach of Stephanie's outstretched arms and shot a look at Loretta.

'Can I touch her?'

'She won't break!'

Carmel leapt forward and collided with Stephanie's desperate embrace, sobbing as her friend continued to utter her name.

'Carmel . . . what's happened . . .?'

Carmel's presence, however, gradually had a settling effect on Stephanie, though she couldn't seem to discuss anything coherently. Carmel looked to Loretta for guidance. 'What'll I say?'

'Just small talk . . . drivel . . . anything. She'll probably flame out again soon.'

Loretta's prediction duly came to pass as Stephanie drifted once again into the land of Nod.

Carmel remained by Stephanie's side for a few minutes. Then she suddenly caught sight of Maria, whom she had rushed straight past in her haste to see Stephanie. She gasped at the sight of the battered commander with intravenous lines and monitors and the enormous chest drain.

'Mother of God . . . Maria!'

Loretta quickly reasurred Carmel. She figured that the young technician could only take so much emotional trauma; it seemed that if anything that the young heroine had been neglected and the effects of her ordeal unrecognised.

'Don't worry. She's recovering. Has anyone told you what happened to her?'

'I knew her face plate was smashed . . .'

'She burst her lung as well. Probably when her suit repressurised. You got her back just in time.'

Carmel appeared drained. She buried her head in her hands. This latest revelation was clearly too much for her. Loretta waited patiently for her to speak and unload her mind, Carmel eventually obliged.

'You mean, Maria could have died as well, if only I hadn't been blown off by that stupid oxygen port. I'd finished. Another second and I'd have moved away.'

'Rubbish!' exclaimed Loretta firmly. 'There's no way that you can blame yourself. There were no villians, Carmel, only heroines. All three of you combined at different stages to save each other.'

'She grabbed me when I was blasted away,' sighed Carmel. 'Then, if it hadn't been for her the tug would have got away.'

Loretta nodded as Carmel debriefed herself, something she obviously had not had the time to do.

'You should see the way she moves in a space suit . . . it's incredible. I always feel as if I'm in a strait-jacket, yet Maria flipped around as if she was in a leotard!'

Loretta decided that it would be therapeutic for Carmel to continue to relieve her mind, so she decided to play psychiatrist.

'What did you think when Stephanie released the tug?'

'I wanted to die. At least I didn't want her to die. Me instead.'

'But without you she had no hope . . .'

'I know, I know. At least I didn't know what to think, or what to do, especially after Maria was hit . . .'

'What you did, Carmel, was to pull off a near impossible rescue. To recapture the tug. Then, according to Adam, cut at least ten minutes off the return journey. My girl you are made of unadulterated raw courage!'

Carmel sniffed, smiled then laughed. Loretta knew that her counselling was complete. She stood up and announced. 'Come over and say hello to Maria.'

Carmel appeared slightly tentative, but Loretta encouraged her.

'Maria,' whispered Loretta, 'Carmel's here to see you.'

In spite of the sedation, Maria's eyes opened instantly. She immediately recognised her rescuer and grasped Carmel's hand.

'Carmel, you saved my life.'

'If I did, it was only because you got smashed up catching the tug,' replied Carmel.

Maria tried to shake her head. 'I was useless after that! I couldn't see. I had pain everywhere. Oh. And then when you took off, my suit slammed into my fanny.'

'I'm sorry about that,' Carmel said apologetically, 'we used to call the tug "the passion killer".'

Maria started to laugh, but she quickly stifled the desire as a searing pain surged through her chest. She gasped instead, turning her attention to Loretta.

'See what she does, always causing me pain.' Maria immediately turned back to Carmel, however, and placed her hand warmly against her cheek and smiled.

'Just kidding!' she uttered as Carmel smiled in response and placed her own hand over Maria's.

'That's enough, you two. If you dislodge Anna's drain

tube she'll kill me!' intervened Loretta.

'Go ahead and dislodge it,' replied Maria, 'it's driving me crazy anyway!'

Loretta shook her finger at her obstreperous patient and led Carmel away.

Shortly after Carmel left, David appeared to find both patients sound asleep.

'It looks like I've missed the action,' he remarked, 'did Carmel help calm Stephanie down?'

'Yes, she did,' replied Loretta, 'and just as importantly, the visit did a lot for Carmel.'

'You mean . . .'

'I mean no one seems to have debriefed her, or even given her a chance to get things off her chest. She even had guilt feelings about the accident.'

'And how is she now, Dr. Freud?'

'She's fine,' replied Loretta, grinning and tossing a rolled-up bandage at David, whereupon it unravelled like a streamer. With the bandage draped across his shoulder, David replied, 'Point taken . . . point taken. And how long have you had these aggressive tendencies?'

'Oh go away, you useless doctor, and let me get on with my work!'

As a tribute to fitness and youth, Maria and Stephanie continued to make rapid recoveries. In fact the nurses knew that they were well and truly out of the woods when they began to make complete nuisances of themselves and refuse to rest or cooperate. Not wanting any late complications, though, David and Anna refused to discharge them from the clinic. Stephanie's memory loss rapidly improved right up to the point just after Carmel's accident. It was then decided to show her the film of subsequent events in an attempt to stimulate her memory some more.

'It's been edited a bit, and the long range shots are a bit fuzzy, but all the dialogue is in,' said David as he set up the viewer. Apart from David, there was an all-female audience, consisting of Loretta and Kate, Maria and Stephanie, and Carmel who had not seen the film of her adventures. The film certainly contained some riveting moments. The camera angle showed the full force of the blast; Stephanie's slalom through the gyrating arms of the DSP also drew gasps. She remembered taking off in the tug, but nothing afterwards. Her eyes widened as she heard her voice announce that she would detach from the tug, so that it may save the others; her mouth dropped as Carmel's hysterical reply echoed about the room. The return journey, of course, had no meaning for her, though she and the remainder of the audience applauded as Carmel neatly dispatched her passengers into the dock.

Apart from any therapeutic value, the film proved a great source of entertainment now that the drama of near loss of life had passed. Whilst the euphoria still ran high, Carmel stood up and announced. 'I've just been reminded of a debt that I have to settle. Maria grab Steph!'

Maria seemed instantly to understand Carmel's intentions and had grasped the bewildered Stephanie and rolled her over before she had time to object. With that Carmel whipped up the loose 'hospital' type gown and brought her hand down firmly on Stephanie's buttocks, leaving a red handprint and a shrieking Stephanie. Carmel sprang back and put her hands on her hips.

'That's one I owe you,' she snarled, 'you little twerp.'

Carmel and Maria then rocked with laughter as did Stephanie, though her guffaws were interspersed with cries of pain as she grasped her posterior. The medical attendants looked on with horror at the treatment of their prized patient.

'Leave our girl alone, you savages,' screeched Loretta.

'Ooh! Look what the beast has done to me,' wailed Stephanie, playing up to the occasion and unashamedly lifting her gown to reveal a crimson replica of Carmel's hand on her delicate bottom. The gathering degenerated into pandemonium as Kate suddenly produced an ice pack and applied it to Stephanie's bruised dignity. Maria suggested that David kiss it better and Loretta suggested Carmel's backside be exposed and retribution administered. David decided quickly to retreat from the scene of crazed females who had decided to indulge in some boarding school-like dormitory ritual. He also decided that Maria and Stephanie's admission to the clinic would be brought to an end. They would probably be far safer back at work.

David returned later to find the nurses in the same wicked mood that had infected the group before.

'Come back for some hanky panky,' tittered Loretta. She further shocked him by lowering her slacks and projecting her rear in his direction.

'I'm off again,' he announced and swivelled around and left to the hysterical giggling of what he had previously thought were his 'professional' colleagues.

Having recovered from their close encounter with death, Maria and Stephanie were quickly absorbed back into the community of the DSP. Towards the end of their recovery, whilst they convalesced, Adam had given the order to activate the ion gun and the slow deceleration of the DSP began. The crew kept a constant supervision of the process, which left little time for socialising, except in pairs or small numbers. Loretta and Kate found themselves seconded to the technical areas, whilst Anna and David occupied themselves in the garden. However, as time went by, it appeared that the deceleration had become a somewhat routine affair and more and more of the crew would be stood down at any particular time.

Loretta and Kate both suffered the same burning desire to discover the true story behind their young ex-patient, but always were rostered on opposing shifts. They both worked with Stephanie at various stages, but the opportunity to discuss personal matters never arose, either due to the presence of other personnel or the pressure of their duties. Both nurses had noticed, however, that on leaving their medical care, Stephanie had resumed a more mature appearance, complete with augmentation of the mammary area. As the opportunity to spend time together increased the two detectives laid their plans.

'What about the direct approach?' asked Kate after some fruitless discussion by the two.

'You mean . . . OK kid . . . the game's up. Tell us the truth or we'll throw you overboard,' replied Loretta.

Though the remark produced some light-hearted relief, it also had the effect of stifling discussion again and they both sat in silence, cramped in Loretta's quarters for the sake of privacy. Loretta eventually attempted to reactivate the discussion.

'Perhaps we're only trying to satisfy our curiosity after all . . .'

'We've said that before,' interrupted Kate, 'and it's true. I'm the first to admit it, but if Stephanie is playing out some elaborate charade, it probably wouldn't hurt her to have someone's confidence. It must be stressful to maintain the pretence.'

'Remember when David said that he would be surprised if someone else didn't know. After all, she must have had help,' added Loretta.

'Anna and David don't appear to have pursued the matter, have they?'

Loretta shook her head. 'They haven't said anything. I suspect they think it is best left alone, which may be the best thing to do.'

'This discussion is going around in circles,' said Kate with a sigh, sounding frustrated. However, Loretta was more determined to get to the bottom of the mystery.

'If someone else knows all about Stephanie, perhaps we should approach whoever it is.'

'Very good Sherlock. Assuming it isn't one of us or Anna or David, and we can't even be one hundred per cent sure of that, so which of the remaining sixteen crew members do we start with?' replied Kate.

'Carmel!'

Kate frowned before she replied. 'For some reason I agree with you . . . but put it into words for me . . .'

Loretta shrugged and continued, 'I'm not that sure that I can. It's a hunch, I suppose. They . . . just seem to have this concern for each other . . .'

'Yes, but that's probably just because of the circumstances. After all, they did rescue each other,' replied Kate, playing devil's advocate, though underneath agreeing with her friend.

Loretta struggled to support her supposition. 'There's just a few things which stand out. Like when Stephanie was prepared to sacrifice herself. Carmel called her a brat . . .'

Loretta tried to think of some other evidence but her mind seemed to dry up. Kate attempted to help. 'I guess you wouldn't smack someone's bum if you weren't close to them . . . but then I guess the techs are a close-knit group.'

Silence took over again as the two mentally sifted their evidence. Then Kate said, 'Well, inspector, with this open and shut case, do we bring in the suspect for questioning?'

Loretta sighed. 'I don't know what we are so worried about. You know what Carmel is like. You couldn't meet a nicer person. The worst we can do is make complete fools of ourselves.'

'And if we do that, we can't exactly leave town,' replied Kate with a laugh. 'I don't care any more. I've just got to know. Let's give her a call.'

Kate had barely finished the sentence when Loretta pressed the intercom whilst she still had the courage.

Carmel responded immediately. 'Hi . . . Loretta!'

'Carmel, how about coming down. Are you doing anything?'

'No. At least I was going around to see Steph in about twenty minutes when she finishes her shift, so I'll come and see you first.'

Loretta turned back to Kate and spoke rather nervously. 'I don't know how I'd handle a rescue or something dangerous . . . I'm shaking at the thought of asking a friend a few questions.'

Carmel appeared within minutes. She wondered why her two friends appeared nervous.

'Sit down,' said Loretta, trying not to sound too formal. Carmel obeyed. Her eyes darted between the two nurses who were both sitting bolt upright. Loretta bit her lip, then decided to throw caution to the wind.

'Carmel, how old is Stephanie?'

Carmel seemed unmoved by the unexpected question and replied immediately, 'Somewhere between twenty-three and twenty-five . . . I think. Why?'

Loretta ignored Carmel's return question and fired off another of her own. 'How old are you, Carmel?'

'Twenty-five. Are you guys planning a birthday party or something?'

Kate entered the conversation. 'Carmel, Stephanie is no more than sixteen. And you're not twenty-five!'

Loretta turned sharply in surprise at Kate's attempt to cast aspersions on Carmel's age as well, but she held her tongue, rightly concluding that Kate was bluffing, though she wasn't sure of her motives.

'I don't understand,' replied Carmel defensively. Kate softened her tone. 'It's OK, honey.'

Carmel interrupted, not realising that Kate had nothing

else to say.

'You're right. Steph is almost sixteen . . . assuming that we are going by Earth years . . . at least she will be in a few months.'

'Fifteen!' exclaimed Loretta, barely able to contain herself. Carmel bowed her head. There were revelations a plenty to come!

'I'm nineteen,' said Carmel looking up slightly defiantly at her interrogators.

It was now Loretta's turn to spring a surprise.

'Who is Gran?' she asked Carmel, taking Kate aback but completely astonishing Carmel.

'You know everything!' gasped Carmel, 'what will happen to us?'

'Nothing . . .' said Loretta reassuringly and flicking her eyes at Kate. The two nurses moved to Carmel's side and linked arms with her.

'Nothing,' repeated Kate with a grin. 'We are your friends, and anyway, seeing we gathered our evidence in the line of medical duty, so to speak, we are bound by the Hippocratic oath, so your secret's safe with us . . .'

'We just thought that you might want to get things off your chest so to speak,' added Kate, 'at least we didn't know that you were involved. We just took a long shot.'

'What made you suspect Stephanie?' asked Carmel.

'Her immature boobs,' replied Loretta. 'But for God's sake, Carmel, will you spill the beans. Our curiosity is driving us insane!'

'Can I get Steph?' replied Carmel. 'She might be off now.'

The two nodded their assent vigorously as Carmel tapped the intercom. Stephanie's cheery face appeared immediately, whereupon Carmel said, 'Hi Sis can you meet me in Loretta's room? I'll explain when you arrive.'

Loretta and Kate stared increduously in reaction to

Carmel's term of endearment. 'Sisters.' They couldn't be. Relations had been banned in selection of the crew.

Stephanie came through the door before they could put their thoughts into words. Carmel rose as she entered and said, 'The game's up, Sis, they know all about us . . .'

The two nurses wished that they did, or at least as much as they had pretended. Loretta set the ball rolling once more, firstly reassuring Stephanie.

'Don't worry, sweetie, your secret is safe with us. Now where did you two space babies come from?'

A look of indignity initially swept Carmel's face in response to Loretta's remark, but then she sighed, relaxed and began her story:

'I'll start about ten years ago. I don't suppose that you ever heard of a famous rescue on an Australian surf beach . . .'

'The guy that saved about a dozen people single-handed and drowned saving the very last one!' exclaimed Kate. 'I read it in *Time* magazine . . . and there was a documentary about it as well . . .'

'Simon Griffin! I remember the name!' exclaimed Loretta. 'Steph . . . you're Stephanie Griffin . . .'

'My Dad . . .' said Stephanie blankly.

'The hell he would be . . .' replied Loretta, barely able to control her emotions, 'And ten years later his daughter nearly repeats history . . .'

'Almost to the day,' said Carmel, 'at least as far as we can tell with time all screwed up?'

'So he was you're father as well?' asked Kate.

'No,' said Carmel, momentarily bowing her head, 'I'll continue the story. Steph lived with her father, and idolised him as did I when I saw him . . . my Uncle Simon . . . we are cousins. I was born in England so I didn't see much of him but when I did . . . well . . . I adored him as well, though neither Steph nor I can remember much now . . .

we were so young.'

Carmel paused for a minute; no one dared speak whilst she formulated her next part of the story.

'Well, as I said, I was brought up in England. My mother was a career woman; she was in her forties when she had me. I don't think that she knew who my father was. I was a bit of a shock. There were certainly no other children, so I was raised by my grandmother.'

'Gran . . .' remarked Loretta, with a satisfied smirk on her face.

'Yes, how did you know about her?' said Carmel, looking puzzled.

'It was Stephanie's first word when she woke up,' replied Loretta with a laugh, 'otherwise I was bluffing, but go on, Carmel, please!'

'Well, going back to Steph . . . her mother died a few days after she was born. She had terminal cancer, they had to deliver Steph prematurely because of her mother's deteriorating condition, so she never knew her, Steph and Uncle Simon were inseparable until . . . well . . . the accident.'

Carmel paused at this point. Obviously an old wound had been reopened. Stephanie merely stared blankly ahead, relieved, it seemed, that Carmel was relating the story instead of herself.

Kate eventually prompted Carmel. 'And your mother, Carmel?'

'I hardly knew her,' came the instant reply as Carmel reorganised her thoughts. 'I haven't seen her for years. As I said, she was a career woman. I still loved her, though, out of respect, so to speak, but it was Gran who raised me. Well, getting back to Steph again ... I'm sorry to chop and change, we've never had to tell the story before . . . have we Steph?'

Stephanie just smiled.

'You're doing a good job, Carmel, just take your time, we're all ears,' said Loretta.

'Well, after Uncle Simon died, Steph was looked after by a succession of people, but none of them really had her interests at heart. They just wanted to bathe in the reflected glory, if you can call it that, and make money out of magazine articles and things like that . . . pathetic stories about a poor little orphan. She was even used in a television commercial. A friend of Uncle Simon's could see what was happening and stepped in. He fought a succession of stupid legal battles and eventually he and his wife convinced the courts what was happening. To cut a long story short, Uncle Simon's friend brought Steph to England and Gran, and me of course,' added Carmel with a grin as she looked at Stephanie. 'So Stephanie and I grew up as sisters; we even call each other Sis. At least we normally do . . . it's been hard disguising it. Uncle Simon's friend and his wife also moved to England. They had two daughters, so we became friends when we were younger, but they moved away, first to London, then they moved to America, so we lost touch. So, as I said before, Gran raised us. We both did exceptionally well at school. Gran always encouraged us, you see. We idolised her. We'd do anything that she asked . . . anything!'

Carmel stopped for a minute and cleared her throat. Kate quickly passed her a drink as if to lubricate the vocal chords of this enchanting story teller. Carmel then continued:

'We were fascinated by the space programme when we were kids . . . I was only thirteen when I decided that I just had to go into space and they were already talking about the interstellar mission. Well, I became obsessed. I was determined to go on it. I didn't care how, I just had to go. Gran had kept all of Steph's legal documents; they were a real education on how to fool the system.'

'But I remember the checks on identity,' interrupted

Kate, 'they were exhaustive, it would have been impossible ...'

'Not for my Sis ...' interjected Stephanie proudly.

'Anyway I did it,' continued Carmel. 'It took a couple of years to set up, and eventually we had some inside help as well.'

Loretta and Kate observed their young colleagues closely; their disguised immaturity seemed more apparent in retrospect, now that they knew the truth. There was more to come, obviously, so the two nurses fixed their gaze on the narrator, who had paused again. Kate took the opportunity to ask a question.

'What did you do about qualifications?'

'It was different in our field,' continued Carmel, 'we were chosen very much on aptitude and ability, whereas I suppose that the medical team at least had to have certificates and so on.'

Kate nodded in reply and Carmel resumed her narrative.

'I was able to impress Jack at one of the interviews and ... well ... I did tell a few white lies about my experience ...'

'But what about Stephanie?' asked Loretta.

'Let me take over, Sis,' replied Stephanie, now eager to offer her side of the saga.

'When Carmel was selected, I was over the moon. I mean I knew that I would miss her terribly, but I was so proud and so was Gran. She helped in the cover-up, or whatever you call it. Gran had a name for it ...'

'Subterfuge,' said Carmel helpfully.

'Yeah, that ...' continued Stephanie, avoiding having to pronounce the word. 'Gran said that she didn't care that Carmel might be breaking the law and all that. Everything went to plan and then ...' Stephanie paused, Kate noted that Carmel had dropped her eyes in apparent anticipation of what Stephanie was about to reveal.

'Gran became ill . . . very ill . . . and she died. She was quite old. I guess that we had thought that she would live forever. So Carmel was lumbered with this orphan kid. We found, though, that Gran had planned things very carefully. We think that she might have known that something was going to happen to her . . . or at least in case it did, she should have some arrangements in place. As I was still under age, she obviously thought that we might be hassled by authorities, so she had secretly arranged for us to move into a flat in a different town. It was all there waiting for us. She also had all these papers to send to my school and other places signed by a fictitious relative exlaining that we were moving and so on, so presumably they were accepted.'

'So you just vanished as it were . . .' remarked Loretta.

'Exactly,' replied Stephanie, 'we were nearly sprung by some reporter, though, he had got hold of my past. We asked him not to divulge anything, but to no avail . . .' Stephanie then gave a short laugh and continued:

'We think the DSP mission saved us. There was a big controversy about the crew selection. It was on the front pages of all the newspapers, plus follow-up articles which forced the "orphan" story into an obscure corner in the middle of the paper. We were gone the next day, anyway, and we never heard any more. It wasn't all that long before Carmel was due to travel to America with some of the European members of the crew . . .'

'I remember . . . I was on the same plane as you, Carmel,' interrupted Kate, '. . . but were you there, Steph?'

'I was, but we didn't travel together. You all went first class and I had to pay for my fare. So I was down the back in economy. Anyway, I could never keep a straight face when Carmel was all diddled up to look more mature. I probably would have given the game away.'

'So when did you make your grand debut into the deception?' asked Loretta, who appeared quite puzzled.

'Ah . . . that's where we needed some help, although the idea had occurred to us . . . especially after Carmel's success. But the crew was all but selected.'

'So who on earth helped you?' asked Kate.

'Can we tell?' asked Stephanie, turning to Carmel.

'I don't see why not,' said Carmel who then continued: 'Do you remember, Kate, the day a group of us went to meet the bigwigs in charge of the space programme?'

Kate nodded in reply.

'Well, I walked into this guy's office. Well . . . you remember how we said my uncle Simon had a friend . . . the one who brought Steph to live in England . . .' Carmel broke into a laugh then continued again.

'Well! There he was sitting behind his desk. He had his head down, looking at my papers, presumably. It had been a few years since I'd seen him, plus I was all tarted up as well . . . so he didn't recognise me. As far as he was concerned I was just another European crew member. Anyway, he started to say something about knowing someone with exactly the same name as mine. At that point I just cracked up completely. I started giggling and said, "Uncle Joe . . . it's me . . . Carmel . . ." '

At this point Carmel dissolved into laughter.

Kate exclaimed, 'Uncle Joe! You're . . . you don't mean Joe Sullivan . . . the bloody director himself . . .?'

Unable to speak Carmel nodded, then regained some decorum and managed to continue:

'He wasn't a real uncle, of course. We just called him that because he had been so good to us. Well . . . he nearly died . . . especially once he found out what I'd done. He said that I would discredit the whole programme. They had already been in hot water about crew selection . . . especially the way they ignored people with qualifications and all those who had been practising hibernation. He said that when my deception came out, it could scuttle the whole mission. So I said, "Don't tell anybody" . . . So he says, "It's too risky and you're too young . . ." So I say, "It can't be too risky if you're in charge Uncle Joe!".'

'I wonder what he is thinking now!' mused Loretta.

'He would think that we're all blown to bits,' replied Carmel more seriously and paused for a minute. Loretta and Kate surveyed the two young imps. What an incredible tale so far. But what about Stephanie? Carmel went on to provide the answer:

'I eventually calmed Uncle Joe down. The poor man . . . I was with him for ages. They kept buzzing him to say that there were others waiting to see him. Then I hit the poor guy with the idea that I wanted Steph to come on the mission as well . . . He flipped! He asked us around to his house that night and refused to say any more. It was really great. We dressed normally and met up with his daughters, Karen and Millie, again. We hadn't seen them for years either. The next day I did Steph up to look older and padded her in the right places,' added Carmel grinning. 'Uncle Joe wouldn't have a bar of it, and after coming around a bit on having me on the mission, said he was having second thoughts.'

'So he changed his mind?' asked Loretta. Carmel nodded.

'Steph won him over herself. She spoke to him in a really mature fashion. In fact, even though I'm older than Steph, I think because of the hassles she had in childhood that she matured very young, at least psychologically . . .'

'Which meant she would fulfill the director's number one criterion for selection,' said Kate. 'She had overcome a crisis in her life.'

'That's precisely what Steph said to him, she showed him something on the computer which really impressed him as well.'

'What was that?' asked Loretta, sounding intrigued. Stephanie said, 'Just a hypothesis regarding the interrelation of mass and velocity near light speed.'

Carmel continued: 'Uncle Joe was able to incorporate Steph's hypothesis into a mission objective, which he really needed at that stage because the programme had been criticised because of lack of real goals. Well, apart from that, with Gran gone, I just couldn't leave Steph behind, so I pleaded with him. He started to relent and allowed Steph to take the aptitude tests. A couple of the original crew selected had dropped out as well, so there was still a chance. Steph passed all the tests with flying colours, and as Uncle Joe reserved the right to hand pick certain crew members she was set . . .'

'But what about the medicals?' asked Kate.

'As you know, the females didn't have to attend the programme doctors, so that provided the opportunity for some more forgery and hey presto! Steph was suddenly a mature woman.'

'Neither of you are mature,' said Kate more soberly, 'but you are extremely resourceful . . . and cunning.'

Carmel laughed. 'Steph had a different surname, of course, and kept her Australian nationality, so no one suspected that we were related. The contraceptive hormone pellets that they bunged in our arms speeded up Steph's development a bit, which helped. Uncle Joe eventually came to the party completely and cut the remaining corners and there we were . . . on board!'

The two cousins grinned at each other like the two naughty adolescents that they most definitely were in the estimation of Loretta and Kate. But who could blame them? They had lost the only person left in their life who had loved and raised them.

'What about Joe's wife and daughters, do they know?'

asked Kate.

'Aunty Gloria found out early on,' replied Stephanie. 'She talked to me for hours, trying to talk me out of it, but I was really stubborn, and in the end, if anything, she helped talk Uncle Joe into letting me go. When they started taking photos of the crew and publicising the departure, they had to tell Karen and Millie. They've been sworn to secrecy.'

'Well, I think you're a pair of brats if ever there were!' exclaimed Kate. 'But what a story. No wonder you both reacted the way that you did when each other was in trouble . . .'

'Even though it meant a smack on the bum!' added Loretta with a laugh. They all joined the hilarity, remembering the pandemonium resulting from the retribution Carmel had taken on Stephanie's rump.

Kate eventually managed to say, 'I don't think I'll be able to sleep tonight after listening to that incredible story. Do you girls feel better for telling it?'

They both nodded in reply.

'Much,' said Carmel, 'it's been hard keeping secrets . . . I know that you probably think that we have been terribly deceitful, but we are not really like that normally.'

'We know what you are really like,' said Loretta reassuringly, 'you are the best!'

'How have you . . . er . . . managed with the men?' asked Kate awkwardly.

'If you mean, have we scored? Carmel has . . . and I haven't,' replied Stephanie.

Kate and Loretta laughed at Stephanie's candour, and Carmel spoke defensively. 'Next you'll be giving a blow by blow description.'

'Spare us the details!' interrupted Kate, 'I'm sorry, I didn't mean to pry. I guess that I was worried that you might have run into romantic problems or something.'

Stephanie shook her head, 'I haven't really felt romantic towards anyone, I mean . . . the guys are all very nice . . . I guess I'm not ready yet for that sort of thing.'

No one pursued the subject any further and in spite of the excitement of Carmel and Stephanie's narrative, weariness overcame the group and they decided to disperse. Before going their separate ways, they had decided to relate the story to Adam and Maria at some stage, as well as confirm with David and Anna that their suspicions about Stephanie's youth were true.

Two days later Kate and Loretta arranged a meeting with Adam and Maria, along with Carmel and Stephanie. The four juniors rarely visited the command centre and gazed around in awe. The area was quite spacious in comparison to other areas, though there was general agreement amongst the whole crew of the DSP that no area could be described as claustrophobic — a fact for which the designers were often blessed.

Stephanie's eyes flicked back and forth between Adam and Maria. They made a handsome couple, she thought. Everyone agreed that Maria was beautiful, both in her appearance and nature. Her body always moved with the elegance of a cat. Her eyes sparkled which, in concert with her permanent gentle smile, must present an irresistable lure to men, thought Stephanie. She imagined Maria at the end of her gymnastic routines, in her final pose with face turned towards the judges, the smile exuding a winning confidence. No wonder she had been so successful. Now, incongruously, this beautiful creature had been secreted away on, of all things, a spacecraft. Maria probably had her own interesting story to tell, thought Stephanie. Her thoughts were interrupted by Maria herself, who broke the silence.

'Well, who is going to tell us what this is all about?'

Her eyes roved back and forth, as she wondered from

whom the response would come. It was Loretta who replied.

'After the accident, when we removed Stephanie's clothes, we discovered that she was . . . er . . . immature, and started to wonder about her age.'

Adam appeared quite stunned at this revelation and replied incredulously, 'How . . . how could you tell . . ?'

'My immature boobs!' piped up Stephanie.

Adam's expression changed now to one of embarrassment, especially as he realised that he was staring directly at Stephanie's breasts, which, to him, seemed anything but immature. Stephanie, noticing Adam's line of sight, said, 'they're padded!' a grin broke out on her face in response to Adam's now bewildered expression. Adam quickly turned again to Loretta for guidance. She obliged immediately.

'Well, for various reasons we thought that Carmel might know something and Kate and I conned her into telling us. Carmel, would you like to take over?'

Carmel nodded and noticed the eyes of Maria and Adam immediately fix themselves upon her. She recounted the story once more, with Stephanie adding bits here and there, and Loretta and Kate making comments along the way. Maria and Adam listened intently, not once interrupting. At the conclusion there was a short silence, which was then broken by Maria.

'Well Captain, are you going to throw the stowaways in the brig?'

Adam laughed more heartily than anyone had ever heard before, then replied, 'They're hardly stowaways. I guess I couldn't ask for two better crew members. Carmel, I wish I'd been a fly on the wall when you broke the news to Joe.'

'The poor man was shocked,' replied Carmel, 'I suppose the whole thing had been a bit of an adventure up until then. Uncle Joe had so many other problems to contend with . . .'

'You have no idea,' said Adam. 'You wouldn't know that the entire crew now on board was nearly replaced by an alternative. The hassles Joe overcame were enormous. Then "his" crew by everyone's estimation back on Earth — has blown up the DSP.'

'Which makes it even more important that we succeed,' concluded Maria. She then asked Stephanie a question that had been gnawing away inside her. 'Steph, what was the hypothesis that you managed to impress Joe with?'

Stephanie blushed, then replied, 'Oh! It had to deal with a fundamental change in a variable. If that variable became unreal . . .'

Maria's eyes widened, whilst the remainder of the group were lost.

'Tell us more,' requested Maria. A fusion of minds was about to occur, it seemed to Adam.

Stephanie took a deep breath and said, 'Well, if a variable in an equation changes . . . that is . . . either becomes large or small, for the equation to hold true . . . it shouldn't become unreal. If it does at any point, then the variable must undergo a fundamental change, be it a sign change from positive to negative or . . .' Stephanie paused and frowned. Maria shot a quick glare at the others. If any of them spoke and distracted the young genius it would be grounds for extermination. Fortunately, no one spoke and Stephanie continued, '. . . it is replaced.'

No one spoke at first. When Maria was convinced that Stephanie had finished, she repeated the final word in the form of a question.

'Replaced?'

Stephanie shrugged and replied as if the answer were obvious.

'Yes . . . if something doesn't work any more . . . you replace it. It doesn't matter if it's a machine or a formula.

After all, we replaced Newton's formulae with Einstein's when we moved beyond certain boundaries, so it's the same situation all over again.'

Adam wished that his co-commanders could have used such concise clear logic as he suddenly grasped the thrust of Stephanie's argument. Maria then exclaimed, 'The note ... to Jack ... it was you ...'

Stephanie clasped her hands together and stared directly ahead at the wall. She then nodded and said, 'I didn't want to have to explain it in detail ... I'm not so sure I believe it myself.'

Maria laughed. 'You have no idea how we agonised over time and motion theories and you had the answer all the time ... even before we left Earth. Steph! You're a genius!'

'No!' exclaimed Stephanie quickly. 'I'm just lucky that I was encouraged a lot at home.'

'You're too modest,' broke in Adam. He realised, though, that Stephanie was embarrassed by adulation and distracted her with another question.

'Do you have any other little gems in that brain of yours?'

Stephanie peered into Adam's clear blue eyes. A reassuring smile occupied his face, which had the effect of relaxing Stephanie. She liked her captain very much; perhaps like a father, she wondered, although she only had child-like memories of what it was like to have a father, and Adam didn't seem to fit that mould. Perhaps like a brother, she reconsidered, though once again, she had no brother with whom to compare him. She suddenly became aware that everyone was awaiting a reply to Adam's question.

'We're in a different dimension,' said Stephanie quickly, as if to make up for the delay in her reply. 'I can tell ... especially when I was outside. I could feel it. I'm sorry, I can't quite put it into words, but we need to be careful . . .'

Something appeared to suddenly come to Stephanie's mind and she quickly snapped a question at Maria. 'Maria did you think that the light beams were bent slightly outside? You know . . . they appeared to arc along the surface of the craft.'

'Yes . . . yes . . . I remember wondering myself . . . Why? . . . Do you have an explanation?'

'Only that it is the craft that is bent, not the light; hence the stress fractures, particularly if we accelerate or decelerate too fast.'

Maria flopped back, flabbergasted. She addressed a question to Adam. 'Do you think that Joe did the right thing in letting this adolescent on board?'

Adam broadened his smile and nodded in reply.

Without any prompting, Stephanie continued, 'To travel at these speeds and in this dimension, the craft needs to be a different shape.'

Five pairs of eyes now fixed themselves on Stephanie in anticipation of another revelation. It soon followed.

'If the craft were circular, and especially if it rotated in the plane of the direction of travel, then the forces would be distributed more evenly.'

No one knew what to say. Eventually the only mind in the group which could match the capacity of Stephanie's commanded its owner to speak.

'Flying saucers!' exclaimed Maria, noticing a smile of recognition appear on the face of her teenage colleague.

12

The speed of the DSP had been gradually whittled down such that it now approached the speed of light, albeit from the other direction. Before the new critical phase of the mission commenced, Adam decided upon an all-crew social event to elevate the spirits. It proved a major success in terms of morale-boosting anyway. A few injuries resulted from over exuberance, but fortunately were of a minor nature.

Carmel and Stephanie's secret was not revealed to any other crew members. The two youngsters soon found themselves absorbed back into the routine of the craft and treated no differently, even by those who did share their secret. Stephanie, in particular, managed to deflect any amorous approaches from her male colleagues, such desires soon being satisfied by more willing individuals amongst the other females of the crew. Carmel and Bud had a steady relationship and Adam duly responded to Maria's charms, much to everyone's approval.

Anxiety grew in anticipation of the transition through light speed. A brief burst of conventional power was decided upon at the critical point and the crew manned identical stations to those they had taken when they had catapulted in the other direction. This time the manouevre was accomplished entirely without incident, much to everyone's relief.

Once back in a familiar dimension the crew of the DSP eagerly trained their telescopes on the surrounding environment. Their theories now became reality, as explained by Alex to the assembled crew.

'We are staring down the throat of Proxima Centauri. We can already make out planets and should have the whole system mapped within twenty-four hours. We are approaching at right angles to the plane of the system, so we are already closer to the star itself than the outermost planet; we are slowing down somewhat to obtain a better look.'

If their previous predicament had made the crew feel a trifle insecure, then their new situation provoked anxiety, particularly as to how they would plan their course of action in this remote world. Adam took over from Alex and explained their new objectives.

'Now that we're here, we plan to see if there is a habitable planet, or one, at least, which might provide us with materials, if we need them. Does anyone have any questions?'

Bud replied to Adam's invitation. 'Any thoughts on a return journey to Earth, that is unless we find the Garden of Eden here and decide to stay?'

Adam smiled at Bud's humour. 'My own thoughts are that we would naturally return to Earth in due course. It really depends on what we find, and of course it's too early to predict at this stage.'

Bud had voiced more or less what everyone was thinking, and Adam gave the expected reply. With that the crew dispersed and returned to their duties. There was much on Adam's mind, however. He had already determined to treat this alien world with great respect. With several things in mind, he arranged a meeting of his co-commanders, plus Carl and Tony, with a view to checking the state of their food production.

'We've been extremely efficient,' stated Carl, 'the worst estimates of wastage were fifteen to twenty per cent per year. We are running at less than five per cent.'

'Everyone is so paranoid about starving,' added Tony, 'so nothing is wasted, plus we have barely touched reserves.'

'So it is theoretically possible to stay locked up in here indefinitely and survive,' said Adam.

'Yes,' replied Carl, 'though I'm sure that you would agree that it would be nice to place our feet on terra firma even if it was inside a space suit.'

'Yes, I know what you mean,' replied Adam, 'even if it is just on a moon or similar small body.'

After some more technical discussion Carl and Tony departed to their all-important gardens and food production areas. Adam then steered the discussion in a different direction.

'I suppose you have all thought of the possibility of us encountering someone or something which is hostile.'

The others nodded and Adam pressed the intercom and summoned Jack and Helen. After their arrival, he repeated his statement and then continued, 'What can we improvise in the way of defence?'

'Are you wondering about weapons?' asked Jack.

'I suppose that's one thing I'm getting at,' replied Adam.

'Well, Cap,' continued Jack, 'as you know, this mission wasn't designed to encounter anyone, and the idea of carrying weapons which might only be used to fuel a mutiny was very strong in the minds of the planners. I'm afraid the most fearsome artillery is in the kitchen.'

'You mean tie a few of Henry's knives to sticks and use them as spears,' said Yvonne with a giggle.

Whilst appreciating the humour, Adam brought the discussion back to order.

'Any useful suggestions?' he said , trying not to sound

deliberately sarcastic.

Helen provided a welcome reply. 'I think our best defence is cloak and dagger. At least initially, on our approach. I mean we can jam electronically and even mask to a certain degree.'

Adam nodded in approval at Helen's welcome suggestion, then said, 'So we really don't have anything offensive as such.'

'We have nuclear fuel, but not the technology to make a bomb or anything like that,' said Jack.

Adam attempted his own humour by replying, 'So it's spears or Molotov cocktails with conventional fuel . . .'

Alex spoke next to reassure Adam. 'Space is too vast to defend, so I dont think approaching a planet should be a problem, providing we do so carefully.'

Adam thought carefully. 'This is all very unplanned, and whilst it seems a golden opportunity, I wonder if we are properly prepared for it.'

Jack replied immediately. 'If we turn around and go back home, can you imagine the powers that be mounting another mission? And if so, when? And probably with a different crew. I think I speak for the crew, Cap, when I say that this is our adventure, or discovery, or whatever you like to call it. Whoever approaches this system will have to face the music, and I'd bet it is wits, not weapons, which will be more important.'

All heads nodded as Jack completed his oration. Even Adam found his head responding to Jack's cold logic.

'Well, let's plan our approach,' said Adam, 'what exactly do we expect to find?'

'This system presumably evolved at the same time as our own,' said Yvonne, 'and we know that galaxies and presumably their individual star systems obey certain rules, so I suspect that there will be more similarities between this place and our own than differences.'

Alex frowned, then added a note of scepticism. 'It does depend on the amount of material condensed at the time of formation and its configuration, though. We may be in for some surprises.'

The others nodded in acknowledgement.

'If we do find a nice Earth-like planet, who gets to visit it?' asked Helen.

'It depends on our technical capabilities . . . the gravity and things like that,' replied Adam. 'Also, if it is Earth-like, there would be parts of it that we probably wouldn't wish to visit!'

'I think it is all speculation until we get there,' said the more pragmatic Alex, 'but if a planet is habitable, surely we should all go, though it would have to be in groups of course.'

'Well, there's nothing else really to discuss,' said Adam, terminating the meeting. With that everyone returned to their duties.

The atmosphere on the DSP hummed with anticipation. The original mission had been a glorified survival exercise and fact-finding task. Now it had transformed into a full scale exploration of another star system. Their previously mundane existence had metamorphosed into a quest with meaning, and whilst anxiety and apprehension ran high, the spirit of adventure more than compensated.

Twenty-four hours later Alex had produced a map of the Proxima planetary system. The co-commanders mulled over it with great excitement. Alex described the main features.

'You were basically right in your prediction, Yvonne. The system bears basic similarities to our own, though the outer giant planets aren't as large as ours — at least there is nothing to compare with Jupiter anyway.'

Alex then pointed to the inner planets, settling on one in particular.

'This one is the most likely Proxima equivalent to our Earth. It's a bit smaller, though it seems to have a fairly large moon. We need to get a bit closer, expecially for spectral analysis.'

'How long to rendezvous?' asked Adam.

'Allowing for braking and a cautious approach . . . about two months.'

Adam heaved a large sigh and said, 'It's all a bit hard to believe.'

The others nodded in agreement.

'Can we prepare a detailed description of our movements since our initial transition past the speed of light?' asked Adam. 'We'll send it back to Earth. Have we enough power to send it that far?'

'Yes,' replied Yvonne, 'but it will be over four years before it gets there.'

Whilst the commanders laid their plans the technicians had much to do, their duties once again taking them outside the craft in relays, especially as they neared their target. After one such sojourn, Helen and Stephanie made their way back from the dock. They chatted about a planned gathering that was to be held shortly.

'I'll be along in a few minutes,' said Stephanie as they entered the hub of the gravitational area, 'I just have something to do first.'

'See you there then,' replied Helen as she set off in another direction.

Stephanie bounded along initially, then settled into a brisk walk as the gravity gradually built up. She eventually reached her quarters and pulled down the top of her suit. She felt hot and sticky, so she pulled out the gel-filled implants which she used to augment the apparent size of her breasts and fanned her chest with relief. Her make-up was then touched up and the bust restored. She rummaged in a small satchel and withdrew a small envelope and hastened out of the door. She travelled in the opposite direction to the place where her colleagues were gathering. Instead she headed for one of the gardens, where she found Anna.

'Steph, I thought you were outside . . .'

'We've just got back. I wonder if you could do me a favour?'

'Of course,' replied Anna appearing puzzled by Stephanie's rather serious expression.

Stephanie produced the small envelope and offered it to Anna. 'Can you plant these? They're sterilised . . .'

Anna took the packet and opened it. 'Seeds?'

'They're flowers,' said Stephanie.

'There's no doubt about you,' said Anna, 'you realise that this is highly illegal.'

'I know. I realise the risk of introducing disease and all that, that's why I had them sterilised before I left. I've zapped them again anyway.'

'Very well, I'll put them in an isolation chamber in Tony's section,' said Anna, remembering a comment that Tony had once made lamenting the lack of romance in the garden, as he put it.

'Thanks,' said Stephanie as Anna pocketed the seeds. She then turned and scurried off to rejoin her friends. She hurried as she approached 'the lounge', as the techs called it, mentally cursing the built-up sneakers that she wore, as they tended to throw her off balance. As she rounded a corner she suddenly caught her foot and stumbled. Alan appeared beside her as if by magic and caught her, thus arresting an almost certain face first collision with the floor. His firm grasp aroused an unfamiliar emotion.

'Gotcha!' exclaimed Alan as he completed the rescue.

With Alan's arms firmly encircling her, Stephanie blushed, partly with embarrassment, but also in response to this strange new emotion. Her heart raced and she was uncharacteristically lost for words. Once restabilised, Alan spoke for her.

'I thought you were going to land flat on your face, Steph . . .'

'I . . . I . . .' she stammered.

Alan slipped Stephanie's arm around his and proceeded to march her forward.

'Hang on to me and I'll make sure that you arrive safely,' he said with a laugh.

The DSP began its final approach towards the Proxima 'Earth'. As predicted, it was smaller than the Earth in the solar system with which they were familiar, but it had a larger moon, which Alex had also predicted. A landing on this moon was discussed, but then it was decided to orbit it instead. In so doing they would study the planet more closely. Orbiting the moon resurrected long dormant feelings of familiarity in the crew after travelling through the void of space for so long. Once the analysis of the planet was complete, Adam assembled the crew.

'It's a different world down there,' he announced as he stood before the giant screen. The latter then lit up with a succession of images, which Adam described in turn.

'There is one enormous land mass and two much smaller, then the rest is presumably ocean with moderate-sized polar caps. The rotation of the planet is different, one day being equivalent to about eighteen hours in our terms. The moon must appear absolutely gigantic on the surface, so they must have some spectacular tides. There is no obvious sign of intelligent life, but we are really too far away to tell for sure. There certainly doesn't seem to be the plethora of satellites that we have around our Earth. Our next step will be to move into high orbit around the planet and then . . . we will contemplate a landing. We can't quite determine the exact oxygen content of the atmosphere as yet, but there is plenty of greenery. Gravity, by our estimates, should be approximately four fifths of what we are used to.'

And so the Deep Space Probe edged its way into orbit around the alien 'Earth'. No one had really come up with a name for the planet; it had come to be referred to as the Proxima Earth in conversation and the term had stuck, except when it was merely called 'the planet'. With more precise detail about the planet, the technicians had busied themselves with the shuttle, adapting it to conform with the demands of the gravity it would face. A closer analysis of the land masses was also prepared, along with a watchful eye for signs of life. Once in orbit, Adam discussed the next phase with his commander colleagues and Jack.

'So where do we aim for, Jack?'

'On the edge of the big continent near the equator, I'd say. There's greenery nearby and some flat areas. There should be water, and even if it isn't drinkable, we can distil the sea water.'

'What about power?'

'We'll use a small nuclear reactor mainly. It's a bit grubby, but efficient.'

Adam frowned. The thought of humans bespoiling a possibly pristine planet disturbed him. However there didn't seem to be much choice. He addressed his next question to the group in general.

'Has anyone found any sign of life?'

'There is some electromagnetic radiation,' replied Yvonne, 'but it's scattered and intermittent. Of course, in this orbit we can't see everything.'

'Nor can we say for sure that there is nothing else orbiting,' added Alex soberly, 'but there doesn't appear to be any complex array of communication satellites.'

'Which means that we shouldn't be blown out of the sky,' replied Adam.

'I guess so,' Alex said, somewhat taken aback by Adam's

military emphasis.

'So when do we contemplate a landing?' asked Adam.

'Give us about seven days,' replied Jack, 'Maria, you will need some time to do our orbital mechanics won't you?'

Maria nodded and Jack continued. 'Then once everything is programmed into the shuttle, we'll need to do a few runs through. Then we can give the all clear.'

With these plans laid, the crew set about putting them into effect. Their situation once again produced feelings of tranquillity, perhaps as a result of orbiting the Earth-like planet with a moon nearby. Stephanie met Anna again, this time in the clinical area. She sat near the spot where she had lain so close to death previously. Anna prepared to insert a new contraceptive pellet into her young colleague's arm, a task that had occupied her for the last hour or so, as the other female crew members had trooped in one by one.

'I suppose I would be cheeky if I asked if you really need this,' said Anna with a smirk on her face.

'I guess I don't . . . at least I haven't up until now,' replied Stephanie. 'But you never know, I guess. And it does make my boobs develop.'

Anna laughed and changed the subject. 'By the way, your flowers are ready. They're beautiful!'

Stephanie's eyes lit up immediately. 'Oh, wonderful!' she exclaimed excitedly. 'If I had anything to do with the planning of this mission, I would have set aside a corner of the garden for flowers. I have always had my own plot at home.'

'I think that the planners wanted every inch for food production,' replied Anna, 'but I'm inclined to agree, especially after seeing yours. It's a beautiful selection. Come and pick them when you're ready.'

Later that day Adam took leave of his command and set out for his quarters. Maria joined him en route and took his arm as they approached their destination. Immediately in front of the door they both noticed a long metal box. Maria recognised it as one of the tech's storage containers. A small tag sat on top with one word written in a neat hand. 'Captain.'

Adam stared at the object until prompted by Maria. 'Go on Adam. Pick it up and open it!'

Adam felt uneasy about the unexpected package, but without comment lifted it up and took it inside and placed it on the end of the bed. Maria plonked herself beside it.

'Someone has left you a present,' she said excitedly.

Adam tentatively lifted the lid of the box as if he were afraid it might explode. Maria gasped and clutched her face.

'*Fiori!*' she exclaimed as if she had discovered gold. Adam just stared at the beautiful floral arrangement. He appeared dumbfounded at the totally unexpected gift. He stood motionless, not really knowing what to do. Maria carefully removed the colourful arrangement. A note was revealed in the bottom of the container. Adam picked it up and appeared even more bewildered. He handed it to Maria, who was still cooing over the flowers. She read the note aloud.

'To our dear captain. May you have safe and happy landings.'

'Who could have sent them . . . and where did they grow them?' said Adam, suddenly finding his voice.

'A secret admirer, it seems. I should be jealous!' exclaimed Maria with a giggle.

'But who?'

'Really, Adam, don't be so slow. Someone has a crush on you, and who is it that develops a crush?'

'You mean . . .'

'There is only one child on board this craft!'

'And only one individual daring enough to flout the rules and grow flowers. I'd forgotten how beautiful they could be . . .'

'So what will you do, Captain?'

'I don't want to embarrass her of course. But it is such a kind thought. Do you have any suggestions?'

'This girl has spent much of her life acting as a woman. Now she has behaved as one her age would, you should respond.'

'But how?'

'The way you feel, of course. You don't have to plan it like a military operation. Just talk to her. Let her be herself for a short time. She realises that our lives are about to change. She probably senses danger on that planet beneath us. She may even feel that she may lose you, as she lost her father.'

Such emotional ramifications of the landing on the Proxima Earth had clearly not occurred to Adam, though he was acutely aware of danger himself; in fact he often seemed to harp on it in the view of his colleagues.

'Do you really think that I am a father figure to her?'

Maria shook her head in reply. 'No, she wouldn't think like that, I know. But you are her security on this craft. If anything, you have probably replaced her grandmother. In fact, Adam, apart from being my lover, you are a natural leader. How often do you hear any discontent on this craft? Never. Did any captain on your ships ever enjoy such loyalty?'

'I think we are a bit more interdependent than the usual ship's crew,' replied Adam modestly, 'we can't afford to argue!'

'Well, I think that you should go to that young girl right now,' said Maria. 'In fact I won't be your lover until you do!'.

Adam laughed at the ultimate but efficient female blackmail weapon and complied.

'Jack!'

'Adam, what brings you to our neck of the woods?'

'I'm looking for Stephanie.'

'You've just missed her. She finished here about ten minutes ago. She said she was going to the garden.'

'Thanks, Jack,' replied Adam and set off again. Jack wore a puzzled look. It was most unlike Adam to go chasing individual members around the craft, but he figured that Adam had his reasons and didn't give the matter much further thought.

Adam entered the garden area, where Anna was on duty.

'Anna! Has Stephanie arrived here?'

Anna appeared defensive and lost for words.

'I know about the flowers!'

'Oh! You do?'

'Yes, don't worry. I presume all due precautions were taken.'

'Of course. I'm sorry, Adam, it's my fault. I guess she struck me at a weak moment and . . .'

'Don't worry,' replied Adam with a reassuring smile, 'if it were anyone else it might be different.'

'That's more or less how I felt. She's down the far end near the isolation bins. By the way how did you find out?'

'The Captain knows all,' said Adam, the smile converting to a wicked grin.

Adam meandered through the greenery and eventually spotted his quarry. He didn't wish to startle her, but in any event she sensed his presence and spun around. Adam spoke quickly to reassure her.

'It's OK, Steph, I've come to thank you for the beautiful present.'

Stephanie wore a stern expression, then dropped her eyes as she replied. 'How did you know it was me?'

'I didn't really, but I had the clever Maria with me.'

'Trust her, she's so smart,' interrupted Stephanie. 'I'm sorry, I . . .'

Adam moved quickly forward and took her hand. 'It was a wonderful thought, Steph. I really do appreciate it.'

Stephanie shrugged. She still seemed embarrassed. Adam tried again to reassure her.

'No one else has given me such a nice present.'

'It was supposed to be anonymous,' said Stephanie.

'I realise that,' replied Adam, 'but I felt I had to let you know how much I appreciated it. It's tough being captain, you know, always having to play a role and never be emotional. One has to constantly say what one thinks is correct, not what one thinks.'

'I know what you mean,' said Stephanie enthusiastically, 'that's how I feel all the time. I just knew that you would understand. That's why I wanted you to know that there was someone on board who cares about how you feel, apart from Maria of course.'

Adam certainly felt out of his depth with this deep and meaningful conversation. Before he could reply to Stephanie further though, she suddenly encircled him with her arms and began to cry. Adam was completely lost for words, but he remembered Maria's advice: 'Let her be herself . . .' He presumed that Stephanie's waterworks were part of the therapy of releasing pent up emotions.

Maria, surmising that Adam may not be equal to the task of dealing with teenage emotions, had followed his trail. Jack wondered whether he would end up giving directions to all the commanders in turn in their quest for his young subordinate. As Adam was about to drown in Stephanie's tears, Maria sprang to his rescue from behind the bushes.

'The captain and a damsel in distress,' she announced melodramatically.

The utterance had the effect of disengaging Stephanie from Adam, whereupon she immediately reattached herself to Maria. The sobbing subsided and a tear-stained face spoke apologetically.

'I'm sorry, I don't know why I did such a dumb thing . . .'

'Don't say such a thing,' interrupted Maria, 'it's a pity we didn't have a bit more romance around here.'

'It wasn't meant to be romantic,' said Stephanie wiping her eyes, 'just friendly . . .'

Maria separated herself from her young friend and held her firmly by the arms. She spoke sternly.

'Look at my face . . . near my eye!' she then released her grip on Stephanie and pulled down her top, revealing a scar above her right breast.

'And see this scar. Do you remember? You saved my life. Now you bring warmth and friendliness to my lover. You are not dumb, *mia piccola* . . . you are an angel from heaven!'

Maria leapt forward and embraced Stephanie and in so doing began to wail and produce her own tears. Stephanie, who had quickly regained her decorum, found herself patting the commander she admired so much re-assuringly on the back whilst staring wide-eyed at Adam.

Meanwhile Anna had advanced out of curiosity and witnessed the soap opera through a strategic gap in the plants. She suddenly became aware of yet another figure behind her. She turned to find Tony looking over her shoulder.

'*E bella!*' he exclaimed, his Latin emotions welling up inside at the scene before him.

Having purged their souls, the individual members of the gathering went their separate ways. Later Stephanie recounted the event to Carmel.

'If I had thought that everyone was going to turn all sloppy, I'd never have done it. Not that I can talk, I guess!'

Carmel laughed. 'Don't worry, Sis. It was a great idea, it probably did Adam the world of good. He always seems so serious.'

'Anyway, I really miss having flowers. It was fun growing them,' said Stephanie.

'Me too,' added Carmel. 'Do you have any left over?'

Stephanie grinned and reached under her bed. She produced a small posy and handed it to Carmel.

'For you,' she said with a grin, 'but don't start snivelling.'

Carmel laughed. 'Who, me? Don't be silly, Sis. But they're beautiful. Here, give me a hug . . . you brat!'

Stephanie found this type of expression of sentiment much more comfortable than the 'adult' variety that she had experienced in the garden. In fact she concluded that circumstances had been coming between herself and Carmel, which had probably led to her feelings of insecurity. Little did she know that a more dramatic separation was soon to follow.

13

'How many do you recommend travel on the shuttle, Jack?' asked Adam.

'Eight,' replied the senior technician, 'perhaps ten at a pinch. But ideally eight. Who will you send, Cap?'

'I will stay behind,' said Adam.

The remark immediately drew protests from Adam's co-commanders, who clearly thought that he deserved the honour of first setting foot on the planet.

'We had it all planned,' said Yvonne. 'With your name, you should be the first man . . .'

Adam interrupted with a laugh. 'Find me an Eve and I might change my mind.'

'Simple, we'll just change Maria's name,' continued Yvonne, taking advantage of the fact that Adam and Maria's love affair was common knowledge.

'No, I'm sorry to explode the myth, but I think it is better that I conduct proceedings from up here. Don't get me wrong, though, I can't wait to get down there. Now let's discuss who else goes.'

The ensuing discussion produced the final crew of eight. Maria was an automatic choice as senior pilot. The others were Yvonne, Bud, Anna, Carmel, Paul, Tony and Loretta.

The landing party was announced, the excitement of those chosen counterbalanced by apprehension as to their fate by those remaining on board the DSP. Carmel and Stephanie discussed the matter.

'I'm sorry you can't come, Sis,' said Carmel, 'you deserve to go more than I do!'

'Nonsense,' replied Stephanie, 'if it wasn't for you I wouldn't even have come on this mission in the first place.'

'And if it wasn't for you, I wouldnt have survived it!'

'No, this is your party, Sis, you can bring me back a flower or a pet or something, just in case I don't get the chance . . .'

'Of course you'll get a chance,' interrupted Carmel indignantly. 'Anyway, what would you prefer? A pterodactyl or a baby brontosaurus?'

Stephanie jumped on her beloved cousin and the two wrestled as best they could, considering that they were partly paralysed by uncontrollable giggling.

The departure time of the shuttle approached and the chosen crew assembled and prepared to board, aided by the technicians who would be remaining. Adam had been to the dock to wish them luck. Then, suddenly, in the command centre an incoming signal appeared. Alex immediately flashed it onto the screen and quickly snapped a call out to retrieve Adam. A face appeared before him and within seconds Adam rushed breathless into the chamber. Alex spun as Adam spoke.

'I got your message. What the . . .'

Before Adam could speak the face on the screen interrupted. Adam instinctively accessed the screen to all parts of the craft.

'May I speak to your commander?' said the stranger.

Adam studied the individual. He appeared middle-aged, with short hair and loose clothing. The accent seemed quite neutral.

Adam replied, 'I am Captain Adam Coleman, Commander in Chief. Please identify yourself.'

'Welcome to our world, Commander. Are you planning to visit us, and what are your intentions?'

Alex studied the screen as Adam formulated his response. The stranger appeared to be seated in some type of communications centre, surrounded by a computerised panel and screens. It was impossible, though, to discern any detail.

Adam spoke again interrupting Alex's thoughts. 'Our intentions are entirely friendly and we do wish to visit.'

'You are from the planet Earth?'

'Yes!'

'We are happy to guide you to a safe landing, Captain. Do you have any weapons that we should fear?'

'No! This is an entirely peaceful mission. We have no weapons of any kind.'

'How many individuals are you sending?' continued the stranger.

'Eight,' replied Adam. 'Can you guarantee safe passage?'

'Of course.'

'How do you know our language?' asked Adam.

'All will be revealed,' said the stranger, in a somewhat patronising fashion. 'I assure you that your crew will be perfectly safe, Captain. I will transmit the landing coordinates. Your lander must leave soon, otherwise you will have to re-orbit.'

Adam shot a look at Alex, hoping for reassurance. A shrug was all that Alex could manage in the circumstances. At least they didn't appear to be dealing with grotesque, hostile aliens, he thought, but the situation appeared all too good to be true.

Adam received instructions from the stranger and Alex set about loading the information aboard the shuttle. Some confusion broke out in the dock at the alteration in plans, not to mention a flurry of animated discussions about the strange transmission. Alex eventually restored order and had the shuttle crew locked aboard in anticipation of departure. Inside, Carmel sat next to Loretta.

'I didn't get a chance to say goodbye to Steph properly. What a shambles.'

Loretta nodded in reply. She gripped Carmel's hand. 'It's all a bit much. Don't worry, Carmel, we'll look after each other.'

Within minutes Maria had guided the shuttle away from the DSP and it commenced its long descent to the planet. Meanwhile Alex fidgeted in the command centre of the DSP.

'That character knows more than he cares to tell us.'

The remark clearly produced a feeling of uneasiness in Adam.

'I know what you mean. Still, I suppose that they are entitled to be wary of us. They don't appear to have anything in space to defend themselves with. We could drop anything we wanted on them.'

Another incoming signal interrupted Adam. This time a different face appeared on the screen, a much sterner face than that which had addressed them before.

The shuttle sped along its prearranged coordinates and entered the atmosphere. The final trajectory mainly took the craft over a vast sea and Yvonne calculated that they would land somewhere in the vicinity of the equator. Silence, broken only by whispers, gripped the crew for most of the journey. Loretta clasped Carmel's hand for most of the trip, the latter turning to smile frequently at her nervous medical colleague, who clearly didn't relish this aspect of space travel.

'Is this sardine can safe?' whispered Loretta.

'Of course it is,' replied Carmel reassuringly, 'I helped check it.'

The final landing approach took them across a vast sandy

beach which bordered a forested plateau, which in turn appeared to slope upward in the distance to a long mountain range. Eventually a long runway loomed before them and Maria guided the craft to a perfect landing. As they eventually came to a halt, Bud piped up. 'I don't think we are exactly in the middle of civilisation!'

They looked about. There were a couple of small hut-like buildings to one side, next to a road which disappeared into the forest. Maria and Yvonne completed their post landing checks and made ready to disembark.

Whatever their overall situation might be, the feeling of exhilaration as each member set foot on this new world defied description. They could be anywhere on Earth; even the vegetation seemed familiar. Each member of the group gazed around in awe. The place seemed deserted until Bud noticed a vehicle emerge from the forest.

'Look! We have company!'

A bus-like vehicle approached them. It moved silently, so they assumed that it must be electrically powered. The crew unconsciously formed a tighter group, as if for protection, as the vehicle neared them. It came to a halt and a man disembarked. They immediately recognised him as the individual they had seen on the screen before departing the DSP. He seemed to wear a plastic smile as he approached.

'Good day. I am Uris. Who is in charge, please?'

Maria emerged from the group. Her eyes penetrated the stranger, who seemed to avoid making direct eye contact as she spoke.

'I am Maria Fontana, co-commander of a deep space probe from Earth.'

Yvonne studied the stranger closely. He appeared overawed by Maria. Most men were, of course, Maria's grooming and demeanour were impeccable, but it was not Maria's physical characteristics, thought Yvonne, that were responsible for this Uris character's behaviour. The man was a jellyfish.

'Please come with me,' requested Uris, the plastic smile reappearing.

The crew boarded the bus, which was steered down the road through the forest. Tony and Anna studied the vegetation intently. The others gazed aimlessly around. Everyone remained silent. They had only travelled a short distance, probably less than a kilometre, when they entered what appeared to be a small settlement. It consisted of a large hut and a few smaller buildings. The area appeared deserted initially, but then they noticed a small group of children in the distance.

Uris lead the group to the main building and ushered them inside. There were several other men, dressed equally as unfashionably as Uris. They were distributed around the room like guards, though they carried no weapons.

'Please be seated,' invited Uris, 'except for Miss Fontana who will accompany me.'

'It's OK,' said Maria, noticing the concerned expressions of her colleagues. She slinked out of the door with Uris, whereupon two guards positioned themselves so as to block the exit.

'Please do not attempt to interrogate my staff,' called back Uris, 'all will be revealed to your commander.'

'Lucky Maria!' murmured Loretta, shuddering at the thought of Maria having to be alone with the creepy Uris. She wandered over to the guards, who immediately closed the gap between themselves.

She spoke in a mocking voice. 'We come in peace. We mean you no harm.'

'And we mean you no harm, Miss,' replied one of them amiably, 'we are familiar with your Earth and its people.'

Yvonne immediately came to Loretta's side and attempted to join the conversation.

'How is it that you know our language?'

'No more,' interrupted the second guard by the door, 'we can say no more.'

Loretta and Yvonne drifted away again. Bud had wandered to a window and peered outside, savouring the brilliant sunshine. He thought that he could hear water in the distance. The remaining seven DSP crew members eventually converged into a group again, and they found their voices.

'What sort of predicament have we got ourselves into?' asked Bud, not directing the question at anyone in particular.

'Well, at least we aren't being chased by headhunters,' replied Yvonne. 'Before we landed, I noticed a larger settlement a few kilometres away and a much bigger runway. I suspect that this is the very fringe of civilisation.'

'I hope Maria is all right,' said Carmel. 'It's weird. These people are just like us. I know that they must have evolved in a similar fashion, but it's hard to believe.'

'Not only that, the forest outside is identical to our own equatorial forests. Even the species are the same,' added Tony.

Eventually Uris returned with Maria, after which he left, taking his guards with him. The crew seized upon Maria. They all sat down whilst she related her story.

'Well, firstly, the reason these people appear so Earth-like is that they are from Earth, or at least are the descendants of Earth people!'

'We thought there must be some connection from what one of the guards told us,' said Loretta, 'but how?'

Maria continued: 'They wouldn't tell me much about any indigenous people, but these people are descendants of individuals who have been snatched by what we would term UFOs! The locals, and those in other nearby star systems, perfected interstellar travel some time ago and naturally visited Earth. They call it Planet of Warriors and regard us as warmongers of the first order.'

'With some justification,' said Bud, 'but why would they want to bring warmongers to their own planet?'

'It's a case of "know thy enemy" you see,' continued Maria, 'they figured that one day we would make it here ... although they weren't expecting us just yet. We've come as a complete surprise ... out of the blue. Anyway, they've bred their own welcoming committee. The individuals here are at least second and up to fifth generation. They know little or nothing of their ancestral Earth, so they are in league with the local power structure.'

'Did they tell you anything about the indigenous people?' asked Anna.

'Nothing. I rather get the impression that they don't know much themselves. The Earth colony occupies the peninsula that we are on now. The civilisations are spread over the large continent and it is forbidden for anyone to visit the two smaller continents to avoid polluting them or interfering in any way.'

'That at least sounds very sensible,' said Tony, thinking of the destruction of the environment on his own Earth.

'So where does that leave us?' asked Bud.

'Ah! We are a grand prize indeed,' answered Maria. 'There have been plans to build up the Earth colony, but the efforts have been thwarted in recent times as they have had increasing problems evading our increasingly sophisticated technology. The biggest snatches apparently occurred during the chaos of the two great wars of the last century, especially in Northern Europe, where millions were never accounted for.'

'But they didn't bring millions,' remarked Anna.

'No. Mind you, I suspect that they would have liked

to . . . More like hundreds. You see, even though they are more advanced in some ways than we are, they are way behind in sophistication, especially in the military sphere. All our wars have put us way ahead. So they see us as a source of great strength which they hope to harness. We are physically stronger as we have developed in higher gravity and we have incredible weapons technology.'

'Aren't they afraid of Earth people taking over?' asked Loretta.

'No, they have no reason. These people were born here and live a normal life, though it's a bit boring by our standards. Their origins are irrelevant; so are the petty squabbles on our planet which their ancestors left behind. Apart from that this is their home, so why go to war over returning to a planet about which they know nothing?'

'So what happens to us?' asked Carmel in a rather small voice.

'Nothing, literally,' replied Maria. 'We're the jackpot . . . medicos, technical people, scientists, plus a sophisticated interstellar craft. Vastly more sophisticated than anything they have and huge by comparison. We are to be assimilated into the community, whether we like it or not.'

'What about Adam and the rest of the crew?' asked Yvonne.

'I don't know for sure, but my guess is that we will be used as hostages and they will be asked to surrender and join us,' replied Maria ruefully. 'We really have fallen into a trap.'

The group became silent as each individual contemplated life on this strange planet.

'It's all very pleasant here,' Loretta said eventually, 'but I resent having my freedom taken away.'

'We noticed some children,' said Carmel, reactivating the conversation with Maria.

'There's a small settlement here. It's main purpose is to provide a reception committee for people like us, but not in such large numbers. It appears that their craft only have room for a few at a time.'

'How come they speak such perfect English?' asked Loretta also returning to the conversation with Maria.

'Actually they speak English and Russian mainly. They figured for many years that it would be either America or Russia which would send the first craft, as they had the original space programmes.

'What about the trees?' asked Tony.

'They're from Earth all right,' replied Maria, 'the whole peninsula has been planted with familiar vegetation.'

'Do we have any idea how many of these Earth descendants are here?' asked Yvonne.

'They wouldn't say. Recent arrivals are apparently kept separate, though, but overall I gather that there are hardly enough to cause a threat.'

'I don't suppose there is any point in making a run for the shuttle,' said Bud.

'It's guarded,' replied Maria. 'We'd be outnumbered, though they seem to have little in the way of weapons. But neither do we, unless you want to throw rocks at them.'

'Are we free to move around?' asked Anna.

'For the time being, only within the clearing. They want us to stay together and cool off, whilst they determine our future. If we behave in a hostile fashion, they will lock us up. For the moment we have to make do in this hut as they are not prepared . . . especially for such large numbers. Of course if Adam and the others join us there will be more. They made a point of requesting that we don't unsettle the people who will assist us. In fact we are forbidden to engage them in conversation until we are given permission . . . except for the children.'

'The children?' asked Yvonne.

'It's probably some sort of psychological softening up process,' said Loretta.

'That was my impression,' added Maria. 'They are probably pawns designed to bring out friendly qualities in order to ease us into their way of life.'

'Well, I don't mind being friendly to anyone,' piped up Paul, 'but it still won't compensate for being under house arrest.'

Further discussion was interrupted by the arrival of food and drink. It was carried in by three women who had the same dowdy appearance as the men, two of whom accompanied them, presumably as guards. The women didn't speak, though they smiled in response to Maria's polite 'thank you.'

'Well, Paul is it up to DSP standard?' asked Anna.

Paul assessed the spread before them. 'Prepared by an expert I'd say. Mmm . . . fresh cheese, we haven't had that for a while.'

Though deflated and dispirited the crew members had retained their appetites and set about devouring the offerings. Later, Carmel and Loretta decided to go for a walk outside. They noticed small groups of children idling about on the edge of the clearing and ambled towards a group of three girls. The children were all neat in appearance, though the girls wore an unflattering tunic-type outfit over short-sleeved cotton shirts. Loretta guessed that they were about thirteen or fourteen.

'Hello!' said Loretta cheerily.

The girls stared warily, their eyes flashing from Loretta to Carmel, who greeted them as well.

'Hello, I'm Carmel and my friend is Loretta.'

Still the girls didn't speak. They're probably not used to captives being so forward, thought Loretta. She turned to Carmel and issued an indirect challenge to the children. 'They don't appear to speak our language.'

'Yes we do!' came the immediate response from the girl in the centre.

Carmel winked at Loretta, acknowledging the clever psychology, then turned to the girl who had suddenly found her tongue.

'What are your names?'

The girl stepped forward. She was thin with long brilliant blonde hair. She was quite pretty, thought Carmel. A smile broke out on her face as she spoke again, a sudden confidence appearing as well.

'I'm Penny, and these are my friends Mara and Elsa.'

'We're pleased to meet you, girls,' said Loretta, 'do you live around here?'

'You come from the space ship, don't you,' said Penny, ignoring Loretta's question. Before Loretta could answer, Penny continued, 'You're going to live with us, aren't you.'

Not if we can help it, thought Loretta. She smiled and said, 'That sounds nice Penny. We would love that, wouldn't we Carmel?'

Carmel received a nudge in the ribs just in case she thought of answering differently.

'Oh yes, it's such a pretty place. You must like it here.'

The three girls responded with a puzzled look as if to say, 'Where else is there to live?'

'We're going to see your space ship,' piped up Mara.

'That'll be nice,' replied Loretta, 'we'll come with you.'

'Oh no! You're not allowed!' exclaimed Penny, her expression changing suddenly.

A woman's voice called the children from the edge of the clearing and in an instant they left. A short time later

Loretta and Carmel noticed a group of about ten children setting off down the road in the direction of the shuttle. Loretta casually walked towards the road, but on reaching it, suddenly found her way blocked by two men.

'Just thought I'd take a stroll, chaps,' she said cheekily.

'It's not allowed!' came a curt reply.

Loretta turned and decided to return to her friends inside. She noticed that the sun was setting. It produced a magnificicent orange glow, which, in turn, intensified the green of the forest. Inside, the shuttle crew sat around in a dejected group and chatted idly. There were a few half-hearted attemps at discussing escape plans, but they all ended with the same conclusion . . . they were trapped. Some time went by when Loretta realised that it was still quite light. She figured that the sun must have set some time ago, so she went to the window. On looking out, she gasped and summoned the others.

'My lord! The moon! Come and look!'

The others quickly joined her and gazed in wonderment at the gigantic moon which filled the horizon. It gave an exotic glow to the atmosphere and kept the crew spellbound for some time, forcing them to temporarily forget their troubles. Eventually their concentration was broken by the arrival of the evening meal. It was every bit as good as the one served earlier and each individual began to wonder whether their predicament was so bad after all.

Earlier the group of children had walked briskly down the road towards the shuttle. They were joined by another group of children. It transpired that this latter group belonged to personnel who had just arrived at the nearby base, seconded, it seemed, to help cater for the DSP crew. They eventually reached the runway where Maria had parked the shuttle. About ten men wandered in an irregular circle about its perimeter. The children stopped and ogled the unfamiliar craft for a few minutes, then began to edge closer. Once within about five metres one of the guards called for them to halt. After staring for a short time, the group of children began to break up. Soon the last few stragglers, which included Penny, decided to leave.

'Can we come back tomorrow?' she called.

'Come as often as you like,' came the disinterested reply.

Not long after the children left, so too did the guards, leaving the deserted shuttle to stand alone, glistening in the moonlight.

The children returned the next morning, their numbers swelled even more by new arrivals, the latter staring open-mouthed at the spectacular craft. There was no sign of any guards, so the more adventurous individuals dared to approach more closely. A few attempted to clamber up the wheel supports when a voice rang out.

'Hey, you kids, off!'

The children turned to see a group of men running towards them. They seemed to have no great fear, but gradually mustered into a group. As the men arrived one of the girls, who was slightly dishevelled, in contrast to the rest, spoke from the group. 'We want to have a look inside, Mister?'

'You can't do that, it's not allowed,' replied one of the men. 'Now how about running along and doing something else?'

Another individual spoke from the group. 'We've just arrived. What do we do around here?'

'Come on, I'll show you,' announced Penny and she led the group away from the shuttle back towards the settlement. As they plodded along, Penny introduced herself to the dishevelled girl.

'I'm Penny . . .'

'I'm Cecily . . .' replied the girl. 'I came with the new group last night.'

'We met two of the Earth people yesterday,' announced

Penny proudly.

'Yeah! What are they like?'

'Really nice. Their names are Loretta and Carmel.'

'Weren't you afraid of them?' asked Cecily.

Penny laughed. 'No, not really, at least we didn't know what to say at first.'

'I don't think that I would like to meet them,' continued Cecily, 'you can't trust them.'

'You've been listening to silly stories,' said Penny. 'Come on, we'll go and see if they're outside.'

A few boys had arrived before the main group. Penny approached them and asked, 'Where are they?'

'They're inside, except for one. They took her away. No, she's coming back now.'

As they looked across the clearing, they saw Maria being escorted back to the main building.

'Did you meet her?' asked Cecily.

'No, but they were beautiful, just like that one. We reckon they must be princesses or something.'

'Princesses?'

'Yes, well they seem to have special clothes, and as I said, they're beautiful.'

Cecily shrugged at Penny's supposition. After waiting patiently, the children were rewarded by the appearance of the shuttle crew, who spilled out of the hut and into the clearing.

'See I told you,' said Penny, still at Cecily's side, 'aren't all the ladies beautiful?'

Cecily just nodded and stood flat-footed until Penny suddenly pulled her arm.

'Come on, there's one we met yesterday.'

Penny dragged the reluctant Cecily in the direction of Carmel, whom she greeted confidently.

'Hello Carmel, this is my new friend Cecily.'

'Hello, Penny, it's nice to see you again. Hello, Cecily,'

replied Carmel.

Cecily stood behind Penny, cautiously peering at Carmel through her hair, which fell about her face. At the same time she clutched the back of Penny's tunic. Penny continued her conversation. 'We went to see your space ship last night and again this morning. A few of the boys started to climb onto it, but then we were all sent off.'

'That's a pity,' said Carmel, 'I'd like to show you inside myself.' And fly off in it, Carmel felt like adding.

As they spoke Cecily drifted away. Penny turned, shrugged and continued her conversation.

'You and the other ladies are beautiful. We think that you must be princesses.'

Carmel stifled a laugh, converting it into a broad smile instead before she replied.

'That's a nice thing to say, Penny, but we aren't princesses, we are explorers.'

'Oh! But you're different to the other people that are usually brought here.'

'Tell me about the others,' said Carmel eagerly.

Before Penny could reply they both noticed two men bearing down on them. The earnest nature of their conversation had attracted unwarranted attention, it seemed.

'I'd better go,' said Penny and skipped away. Carmel glared at the men who curtailed their advance and ambled back towards the edge of the clearing.

'Damn!' muttered Carmel, just as I was about to get some information. As she walked back to the hut, her frown was soon replaced by a smile.

'Princesses!' she exclaimed and chuckled to herself. She approached Yvonne and recounted her conversation. They both laughed at the royal status with which they had been endowed.

'You should have strung them along,' said Yvonne.

'I should have,' replied Carmel. 'It's funny, but I have a hunch that those children might be able to help us somehow.'

14

The stern face on the screen spoke as Adam and Alex watched grim-faced.

'Your shuttle crew will be taken into protective custody when they land. A craft will arrive shortly to transport the remainder of your crew to our space station. Do not attempt to resist and ensure that all remaining members of your crew leave your craft. You will not be harmed if you cooperate.'

The face disappeared. Almost immediately Alex exclaimed, 'The space station! It's materialised out of nowhere!'

'It must have been masked, or hiding on the other side of the planet,' said Adam. 'Damn. We've stepped straight into a trap. We have no choice but to comply. They have the shuttle crew as hostages.'

'They may have other tricks up their sleeves as well,' added Alex.

'I'd better assemble the crew,' said Adam. He contacted Jack and informed him of the situation. He had no sooner finished the conversation when a message came through that the alien transport vehicle had arrived.

Ten armed men came on board. One immediately accessed the DSP personnel files, which scuttled any plans Adam may have had to hide anyone on board. The transfer was anything but orderly. The DSP crew were rounded up in separate groups and placed in different sections of the transport vehicle, which was quite large. Adam and Alex were the last to be placed on board. They heard the leader of their captors report, 'We have them all. They all match up against their personnel files.'

Adam and Alex stayed together for the journey. They were not to see their colleagues for some time.

'They've probably transferred all the personnel information on each one of us,' said Alex in a low voice, 'that's why we have been divided up.'

Adam nodded in reply. He felt apprehensive for his crew and what they might be used for. He hoped that, being all technically trained, they would be treated with respect. It didn't seem too long before they arrived at the giant space station and docked uneventfully. The crew remained fragmented. Adam and Alex remained together. They had no knowledge of what had happened to the others. The two commanders found themselves being escorted to a very sophisticated command centre. The chamber was circular with personnel distributed around the periphery, batteries of screens and data banks lined the walls. The centre of the chamber was lit more brightly, and like a king on a throne, sat the owner of the stern face who had last communicated with them on the DSP. He remained seated and addressed them.

'I am Anderson. I am pleased that you transported your female commanders to the surface. Women irritate me.'

A raving chauvinist, if ever I saw one, thought Adam.

A pompous upstart, thought Alex.

Both remained silent.

'Some of your crew will be sent down. The remainder will remain on board the station and assist us, continued Anderson, placing his hands behind his head and leaning back. He looked away as he spoke again. 'I don't know what use I will have for two ex-commanders . . .'

Alex bristled. Adam could sense his ire and grabbed him by the arm as he answered Anderson. 'I dont know who you are or what your game is, but we are not your pawns, and I warn you to treat our crew with respect.'

Anderson made a sneering sound and spat back a reply. 'Respect . . . I can treat you anyway I like ex captain . . . and there's nothing you can do about it.'

Alex was tempted to answer, but he found himself restrained by Adam's grasp again.

'Take them away,' commanded Anderson waving in an airy manner towards an exit. Adam and Alex soon found themselves in a small room behind a locked door. They spoke in whispers.

'Try not to react to him, Alex,' said Adam, 'I suspect that the intimidation is just part of a softening up process. It's a typical piece of military strategy to demoralise the opposition . . . the first stage in brainwashing.'

'I understand,' replied Alex, nodding. 'It irks me, though, to think that such a dickhead can get the better of us.'

'He's won the first round,' said Adam, 'but the fight's only just begun. Remember what Jack said about using our wits.'

'Yes, good old Jack, I'll bet he has morale well and truly under control.'

'What do you make of these people?' asked Adam. 'They don't exactly appear alien.'

'No,' replied Alex, 'they're from Earth. I don't know how they might have got here, transported, I suspect. We can't be the only ones that have unlocked the secrets of interstellar space travel.'

'I see your point,' replied Adam. 'If that's the case, they could have been here for generations.'

'Quite true,' said Alex.

'I think the best plan is for us to go along with them

and hopefully discover a chink in their armour,' continued Adam. 'They can't be perfect.'

'No, but there will be a problem if we are split up and farmed out all over the place. Especially if we are going to mount any sort of rescue.'

Adam thought for a minute before continuing the discussion.

'Let's just keep our eyes open. We'll have to rely on luck coming our way. We've already got ourselves out of a few jams.'

However, Adam and Alex had little opportunity to expand their knowledge over the next twenty four hours. They were very much confined to quarters, as were the remainder of their colleagues imprisoned on the space station. Like the rest of the crew on the surface of the planet, frustration and boredom began to infect their minds. Yvonne and Maria discussed the problem.

'I think that they are going to bore us into submission,' said Maria as she and her co-commander sat on the steps of their billet.

'I'd still like to have a go at getting away in the shuttle,' said Yvonne.

'We'd have to wait until they dropped their guard,' said Maria.

At that point the grinning Uris appeared. He stopped about ten metres away and called to them. 'Some of your colleagues will be joining you later.'

Maria and Yvonne stood bolt upright. Maria called after him, 'What do you mean?'

But he was already walking away and ignored further exhortations from both Maria and Yvonne for more information. Loretta heard the exchange and hastened over. 'I wonder what he means . . . ugh . . . Doesn't he give you the creeps!'

The other two nodded in agreement. About two hours

later though, the vehicle which had transported them from the shuttle was driven off down a different road. It reappeared late in the day. The shuttle crew quickly recognised the occupants as they disembarked. Carmel searched in vain for Stephanie; instead she saw Carl, Kate, David, Henny and Gerda.

The incumbents rushed over to meet their colleagues. Carmel hugged Kate and asked in desperation, 'Steph . . . where's Steph?'

'The others are still on board a space station, honey.'

In order to prevent a multitude of individual conversations, David called everyone's attention and explained what had happened.

'Just after you all left in the shuttle, we received another transmission and a huge space station materialised from nowhere. It sent a large transport vehicle over and took us all off.'

'Are you sure everyone went?' asked Maria.

'Yes, they accessed our personnel files to make sure that no one hid or anything like that. We were separated into groups. We didn't even see each other on the trip over. I know that they plan to keep the techs up there. We don't know anything about Adam or Alex.'

Carmel's heart sank. The thought of Stephanie being a prisoner or slave on some alien space station for life terrified her. Kate sensed her fear, as did Loretta, and the two nurses immediately moved to her side.

'Did you find out anything about these people?' asked Maria.

'Nothing!' replied David.

'Our lot down here have been a bit more open. Let's all go inside and we can fill each other in properly.'

'The two groups exchanged information, the new arrivals explaining the chaos as they were pressganged off the DSP.

'We had just been toying with the idea of getting hold

of our shuttle and making a run for it,' said Maria in conclusion, 'but I guess that's the end of that idea.'

Whilst the expanded group of DSP crew members held their conference a group of hopeful children waited outside. When no one appeared, they eventually gave up and wandered off, resolving to return again the next day.

A small group of them returned early the next morning and began to play around the edge of the clearing. Carmel had been unable to sleep and rose early, thinking that a chat to the effervescent Penny might cheer her up and take her mind off Stephanie. Loretta noticed Carmel's restlessness and followed her soon after. However, Penny was nowhere to be seen, the children seeming unfamiliar. Carmel was not in the mood to strike up new friendships and sat on the ground a few metres from the steps. She then noticed the dishevelled girl by herself on the opposite side of the clearing to the other children. She was aimlessly kicking a stick along the ground, occasionally looking in Carmel's direction. Carmel sighed and stood up.

'Perhaps I should make an effort,' she muttered to herself.

She started to walk towards the girl, but the latter immediately moved away and Carmel stopped. By this time Loretta had come up behind Carmel and had noticed her intentions.

'She's a funny one, Carmel.'

'She sure is, not like the others. I was going over to be friendly, but she spotted me and moved off.'

'I noticed,' said Loretta.

They stood there for a minute, then Loretta said, 'Come on, I'd like to see what makes her tick!'

They chose a circuitous route as their approach, so as not to appear too threatening.

'How old would you say she is?' said Carmel.

'About thirteen or fourteen,' replied Loretta. 'It's a bit

hard to tell with her hair all over the place. Ugh . . . I'd like to get hold of it and tie it back.'

'Poor kid,' said Carmel sympathetically, 'she looks like a bit of a waif compared to the others.'

They gradually drew nearer to their target, the stealthy approach apparently not noticed by Cecily. She seemed to see the two crew members when they were almost upon her and instantly turned her back. Undaunted Carmel addressed her.

'Hello! It's Cecily, isn't it?'

Cecily kept her back to Carmel and Loretta, but she turned her head slightly and pulled her hair away from the side of her face which faced them. The words that she spoke would be long remembered.

'Hi, Sis! Nice disguise, huh . . .!'

Carmel choked to prevent herself from crying out. She shook with emotion and her hand involuntarily darted towards the grinning figure, but she was shrugged off immediately.

'Get away, silly! You'll give the game away!'

Loretta, whose mouth had dropped open in complete disbelief, managed to speak.

'My God, Stephanie,' she hissed, 'how, on earth did you pull this off?'

Stephanie grinned coyly.

'I stowed away on the shuttle. I've been here all the time.'

She dropped her eyes and turned away, then pretended to move off. Carmel and Loretta followed her, attempting to appear casual, which was extremely difficult for them given the extraordinary revelation.

Carmel asked the burning question. 'But how . . .?'

'It's a long story,' replied Stephanie. 'I've been back to the shuttle at night, the guards are pathetic. I'm afraid we have a few problems on our hands!'

Loretta snorted at the gross understatement.

'You're not kidding, we've all become bloody hostages!'

'Except for me!' said the grinning Stephanie. 'Are we being watched?'

'No,' replied Carmel, 'I think that we are up a bit too early for them.'

'The DSP's deserted,' continued Stephanie. 'I found out from the shuttle's computer. Everything's on automatic!'

'Yes, the others were all captured shortly after we left and transported to a space station. Then some were sent down last night,' said Carmel. She gasped and continued, 'But wait a minute . . . The aliens checked all the crew's ID codes and personnel files. They must know that you are missing!'

Stephanie moved away and kicked her stick along the ground. Carmel and Loretta noticed that some men had just entered the clearing. They waited a minute before casually following Stephanie, who carefully looked about before speaking again.

'I smelt a rat when that transmission came through. I thought to myself, What's an Earth guy doing here . . . and speaking perfect English? . . . And I noticed a computer in the background. Same configuration as the IBM I trained on. It was all too impossible to be true. That is, to expect all that to have evolved on another planet. Whilst Adam was changing the plans, I knew that was my opportunity to disappear!'

'Disappear?' questioned Loretta looking quite puzzled.

'Yes, well, you remember the confusion as the shuttle crew were preparing to leave?'

The other two nodded.

'More like chaos,' said Carmel.

'I accessed the ID codes and . . . well I wiped mine off . . . so I didn't exist any more. Then I slipped into the shuttle amongst the confusion and hid in the reactor chamber, as it has to be kept pressurised.'

'And I was looking for you to say goodbye,' sighed Carmel.

'Sorry, Sis. Anyway, after you all trooped out and were taken away, I waited until night, then all these kids came along. That's when I got the idea.'

'What idea?' asked Loretta, although she presumed the answer.'

'To pose as one of them. I cursed that damned moon, though. No such thing as a dark night on this planet. But the guards wandered off anyway, and so did I! I hid in the scrub for a while, then I raided a house in a settlement nearby for this get up. My hair was pretty messy by then, so I dragged it over my face . . .'

'You look disgusting!' interrupted Loretta with a laugh.

'I bet I do,' replied Stephanie. 'What I'd give for a good wash! So, anyway, there are new kids arriving all the time. They belong to new personnel who have been brought in to look after you lot, so it wasn't too hard to pass myself off as a new arrival.'

'Any other little gems?' asked Loretta.

'Oh yes! The kids carry these computerised ID cards. I nicked one and broke into that office over there and made myself a copy. The security's really slack!'

'They're probably not used to spies like you slinking around in the night,' said Carmel.

'No! But I also accessed all this info off their computer. They don't even have any security codes, they must be really hopeless. So I'll bring a chip from the shuttle tonight and then dump it all in the shuttle's computer. It's got all the guff about a space station, communications and God knows what else. When the right time comes, I'll really be able to stuff them up good and proper.'

Loretta and Carmel were speechless. Stephanie seemed ready and equipped to stage a one person war. The three suddenly realised that they were being watched. Stephanie dropped her head and crossed in front of the other two. Carmel noticed a grin as Stephanie spoke through the tangled hair.

'There's a nice clearing behind you in the bush. Perfect spot if you want some hanky panky.'

'Really!' exclaimed Carmel, but Stephanie had stalked off in an apparent huff. Loretta and Carmel quickly strode back to the hut, sucking in their cheeks as they went. They burst inside and dissolved into uncontrollable laughter, stifling the sound as best they could so as not to disturb the others. As their spasms subsided, they went to the window and observed the irrepressible Stephanie playing tag with a couple of boys. The sight of Stephanie leaping around like a grasshopper reactivated their laughter. They went back to the door and ran around to the back of the hut and spent the next twenty minutes trying to recompose themselves. Even then it would take another hour before they became completely sober and were able to analyse the situation more pragmatically.

'I couldn't sleep last night, I was so worried about her,' said Carmel shaking her head. 'Then she pops out of nowhere!'

'She's unbelievable,' added Loretta, 'but I suspect that she learnt a few tricks from a certain cousin!'

'And a certain grandmother,' said Carmel with a laugh. 'She never had much time for authority . . . at least not for its own sake.'

'I suppose that we should let Maria know,' said Loretta.

Carmel suddenly became cautious and Loretta sensed the wisdom of an experienced practitioner in the art of deception.

'We need to be careful. The less people that know a secret the better.'

'But we can trust Maria,' said Loretta.

'Yes, of course. It's hard to put into words, they have

been interrogating her every day.'

'You surely don't think that they would torture her or anything like that,' replied Loretta, sounding shocked.

'We really don't know what we're up against,' said Carmel and to Loretta she suddenly sounded very mature, well beyond her age. 'These people look like hicks, but there's a much more powerful organisation behind them. We can't even believe what they have told us. We are completely at their mercy and Stephanie is our only lifeline.'

'So what do we do?'

'I agree that we have to tell the others at some stage . . . obviously. It's a matter of when. But I also realise that we can't leave it too long. Someone is bound to wake up to Stephanie sooner or later, especially in a small community like this.'

'I guess we need some advice,' sighed Loretta.

'What we need is information,' said Carmel. 'You can't plan anything until you know exactly what you're up against.'

'Why don't we wait until tomorrow then,' said Loretta reassuringly. 'We can sleep on it, and Steph might have some more information for us as well.'

Carmel nodded in accordance. 'Yes, hopefully one night won't make any difference.'

That night, whilst Carmel struggled to fall asleep, Stephanie had slipped into a nearby communications building. Over the next few hours she quietly pilfered data from the computer terminal, crouching so that she would not be seen if anyone happened to come by. However, only the hut where the crew slept was guarded, as the captors were totally unaware of the maverick who had slipped into their community so cleverly. Stephanie worked unrested for several hours, stopping only for brief excursions to a window to check her surroundings, then returning to her task. The glow of the monitor illuminated her grubby cheeks and matted hair which fell about her face. This bore an expression of total determination and intense concentration.

She carefully placed the invaluable information into a pocket in her tunic and quietly edged out of the building and was soon making her way through the forest. Eventually she arrived at the runway where the shuttle sat dormant in the moonlight. After a quick check for guards, she stole across the open ground and entered the shuttle on the far side, hoping that no one had been stationed inside. Her fears were unfounded and, having checked the interior, she started the second stage of her night's work and began to load her stolen booty into the shuttle's computer. This became a time-consuming task, but urgency banished any desire to sleep, at least until she had at last finished. Exhaustion hit her like a brick wall and she flopped back, intending only to close her eyes for a minute.

A deep-seated instinct forced her eyelids apart and she dragged her reluctant body into an upright position.

'I mustn't sleep here,' she muttered aloud, 'I'll never wake up in time.'

She felt wretched as she stumbled to the exit and hauled herself out and dropped to the ground. She landed awkwardly and took the weight of the fall on her right knee, stifling the cry her mouth wished to expel. She lay on the ground for a few seconds. Still there was no one to be seen. She was soon back in the safety of the forest and headed for the hideaway she had prepared for herself. Fatigue dominated her feelings of dirtiness, itchiness and the pain in her knee, though before descending into a coma-like sleep, she muttered, 'Ugh . . . why didnt I ask Carmel for some soap?'

She awoke with a start. It was daylight and she fumbled under the tunic for her watch, which she had attached around the side strap of her knickers in order to keep it concealed from unwarranted attention. After making the appropriate calculation to local time, she exclaimed, 'It's ten . . . damn . . .!'

She leapt to her feet and made for the settlement, brushing away dirt and twigs as she went. As she approached she noted most of the crew in the clearing and a considerable number of children, more than previously, had struck up conversations with crew members.

Carmel had been on the look-out since early morning. She had long since passed the stage of being worried, despair and fear for her cousin's safety being the horrible substitutes. For the last half hour she had clung to Loretta.

'Something's happened. I'm worried . . .' she kept repeating.

Loretta suppressed her own fears in order to reassure Carmel.

'She must have her reasons. Perhaps she doesn't want to appear too obvious.'

Carmel suddenly applied a vice-like grip to her colleague's arm and hissed. 'There she is!'

'Slow down,' replied Loretta as she felt herself being hastily dragged away.

They approached cautiously, camouflaged to some degree by all the activity in the clearing. The cheeky grin with which Stephanie had greeted them the day before had vanished. Carmel spoke in a gasping manner.

'I was worried about you, Sis . . . Holy Mother, you look terrible!'

'I had a busy night,' said Stephanie, sounding slightly sullen. 'I'm so filthy, I forgot to ask you to try and get me some soap, and something to eat if you can. I've got stomach ache from eating berries.'

'What about water?' asked Loretta.

'There's a lovely stream nearby,' said Stephanie, a faint smile appearing on her face. 'I'm dying for a decent wash. I don't care if I cause pollution, I feel disgusting!'

'I'll get a parcel of things for you,' said Carmel, sounding concerned. 'Where can I leave it?'

Stephanie cautiously looked behind her and answered, 'Just behind the tall tree directly behind me will do. I'll pick it up tonight if I can, but don't take any risks.'

'I'll get it there, Sis . . . by hook or by crook.'

'Any news?' asked Stephanie.

'Nothing,' replied Loretta.

'I've loaded all the information,' said Stephanie. 'It took me all night, I'm sorry . . . then I overslept.'

'Don't apologise,' said Loretta firmly. 'Take a night off tonight and get some rest. Hullo, here's trouble!'

A group of men had moved into the clearing and were dispersing the children and motioning to the DSP crew to return to the hut. Having been momentarily distracted, Loretta and Carmel turned back to find that Stephanie had evaporated into thin air. They stared at each other open-mouthed, then quickly returned to the hut to avoid any undue attention from the guards. As they approached the door, Maria greeted them from the steps.

'You two seemed to be having an earnest conversation.'

Carmel turned to Loretta, who was squinting at her in an attempt to glean her thoughts. Her face remained expressionless as she answered. 'Maria, can Loretta and I talk to you about something later?'

'Of course,' came Maria's predictable reply, 'whenever you like.'

They were to be denied access to Maria, however, as the latter was soon escorted away once more. To make matters worse, the crew was to be confined for the rest of the day.

'How am I going to get some things to Steph?' whispered Carmel to Loretta.

'Not very easily. Especially with all those goons out there!'

They stared at the clearing through a window. The guards had assumed a greater presence than usual. Loretta thought for a minute, then said, 'Perhaps we will have to wait until tomorrow.'

She knew immediately that she had said the wrong thing as Carmel's eyes flashed at her. 'We can't, we just can't! We need a diversion. I wish Maria would come back. I wish I'd told her now. Whatever are they doing with her?'

As Carmel's words tumbled out, Loretta began to think. Eventually she shared her ideas.

'I take it, when you say a diversion, you mean some sort of commotion to distract the guards.'

'Yes, but they all need to be distracted for long enough for one of us to plant something on the far side of the clearing. It would be near impossible, and if we got sprung it could blow Stephanie's cover.'

'We need an excuse to go to the edge,' said Loretta, 'and a good distraction.'

Carmel remained silent. She sensed an idea germinating in Loretta's mind.

'Sex!' announced Loretta bluntly.

Carmel appeared horrified. 'Sex? You're not suggesting we try and seduce . . .'

'Not that type of sex,' interrupted Loretta with a laugh. 'I mean to flaunt it, not do it!'

'Just exactly what do you have in mind?' asked Carmel suspiciously.

'A bit of fun,' replied Loretta. 'Let me explain: one thing that vegetarian diet, over the last year or so, has done for us has been to give us nice bodies.'

'So you want us all to parade naked across the clearing?'

'You're getting warm,' said Loretta. 'What I have in mind, is a bit of make-believe skylarking. It will provide the excuse to run around and make the drop before the guards have much time to do anything about it. First we need some recruits.'

Carmel still appeared mystified, but she was prepared to support any plan which would help accomplish the objective.

The afternoon wore on and still Maria did not return. The guards had annoyingly remained, though they tended to congregate near the road which led to the shuttle. To them all appeared quiet inside the hut where the crew were confined. The tranquil scene was suddenly transformed as the door of the hut was flung open to a loud whoop, shattering the peace.

The guards stiffened in response to the sound. Then Bud and Paul descended the steps, issuing yells of apparent delight. Paul immediately headed in the direction of the exit road; Bud veered laterally towards the edge of the clearing.

As the guards attempted to digest what was happening, Carmel and Gerda burst from the door of the hut. Each was clad only in a T-shirt and knickers, Gerda's attire, in particular, leaving little to the imagination. Bud and Paul both waved a pair of slacks as they ran, which one might correctly surmise belonged to the underclad females who were attempting to retrieve them from the escaping thieves.

Paul ran a zig zag course, though continuing more or less in the direction of the guards. He suddenly appeared to stumble and then wriggled to one side, causing the pursuing Gerda to overshoot slightly. She stopped and bent down, attempting to grab the end of her slacks, and in so doing gave the guards a generous eyeful of her near naked posterior. Paul, however, whipped the elusive apparel from her grasp and jumped to his feet. Gerda dropped onto all fours in frustration and shrieked, maintaining the pose for a second and gaining maximum attention from the onlookers. She then rose and continued the pursuit, issuing loud curses in the process.

Meanwhile Carmel had pursued Bud in a similar, though less erotic manner, towards the edge of the clearing. As the male crew members neared the forest, they suddenly flung the girls' slacks into the scrub. The guards were definitely more preoccupied with the two actors before them — namely Paul and Gerda — who had come within a few metres of them. Paul dissolved into laughter after jettisoning his stolen booty, whereupon Gerda came up to him and commenced attacking him. Still laughing, Paul grasped her T-shirt, and in the ensuing struggle he deftly slipped it over her head. Gerda's breasts spilled out in their sizeable naked glory. She screamed at Paul and broke away, then stalked into the edge of the forest and retrieved her slacks. As she did so the guards were vaguely aware that Carmel was just exiting the forest with hers, though she at least hadn't lost her shirt.

Bud and Paul had turned and were running back to the hut, Paul still clutching Gerda's top. Both girls set off in pursuit once more and within minutes the sudden pandemonium had ceased, though the guards were vaguely aware of the sounds of animated voices coming from inside.

The guards appeared dumbfounded. One eventually spoke. 'What should we do about that?'

'Nothing!' came a curt reply from an individual who had obviously been entertained. 'With a bit of luck, they might do it again!'

Unfortunately there had been other spectators, at least to the concluding moments of the performance. They consisted of Uris and two other guards who had been escorting Maria back to the hut. As the door slammed behind the frolicking foursome, Uris snapped, 'You will be brought back in one hour, Commander, for an explanation of this behaviour.'

Maria shrugged. She was as mystified as Uris, though highly amused. The fact that Carmel was involved, however, set her thinking that there was more to the charade than met the eye.

Inside the hut the remainder of the crew observed the four renegades with puzzled expressions. No warning had been given. Carmel and Gerda had voluntarily disrobed and then, before anyone knew it, the act was underway. The breathless participants now cackled excitedly, Gerda's guffaws interspersed with grimaces of pain as she clutched her bust.

'Ooh! Running without a bra is murder!'

'Here . . . ' said Carmel, reaching under her shirt and undoing the underwear which encircled her own chest. 'It served the purpose perfectly. Do you want me to wash it first?'

Gerda laughed and replied, 'I don't care! All right, what's everyone looking at?'

'Your chin!' replied Paul, barely able to control his mirth. The proceedings came to an end as Maria flung open the door of the hut and appeared in the doorway. They all turned in anticipation.

'I'm glad to see you're keeping yourselves amused,' she said, breaking into a laugh.

'Of course,' replied Loretta cheekily. 'By the way Maria, you're next!'

'They'll never let us go if we start putting on a show for them,' said Anna.

'They didn't find the show very amusing,' said Maria more soberly. 'You're tricks have earned me another visit to headquarters in an hour to explain! So can someone tell me what I'm supposed to say?'

'It was my idea,' said Loretta immediately. 'Carmel and I were talking about ways of distracting the guards. If the need arose, we just wanted to see how easy it was . . . '

'It was a bit vulgar,' replied Maria. 'I take it the idea was to get them to concentrate on Gerda and Paul?'

'Yes . . . and it seemed to work.'

'I'm not surprised,' said Maria with a smirk. 'Gerda, you deserve a medal of honour for bravery beyond the call of duty!'

Gerda, now dressed, replied, 'It was worth it just to see the looks on those guards' faces. Next time I'll do a cartwheel.'

'I hope that you won't have to repeat the performance too often,' said Maria, 'or perhaps we could take it in turns. But only if you guys take your clothes off as well.'

Maria promptly ended her involvement in the banter. She clearly had other things on her mind and she pulled Yvonne aside for a private discussion.

'How did it go?' asked Yvonne.'

'They just keep on and on,' replied Maria with a sigh. 'They demand that I divulge all that I know about the operation of the DSP and the state of scientific development back on the real Earth, and they refuse to let anyone join me during the interrogation.'

'They probably think that it's easier to wear one person down. How are you holding up?'

Maria laughed before replying, 'I had tougher competition at the Olympics.'

'Yes, but if they're desperate, they might resort to something horrible like torture!'

Maria made light of Yvonne's suggestion.

'I can handle that . . . you should have met some of my coaches!'

Time passed quickly and soon Maria found herself being escorted back to the main building in the nearby complex. Once again she faced Uris and two familiar offsiders. The false smile that had initially dominated the face of Uris had gradually faded through successive interviews. Maria's unshakeable confidence had steadily eroded the dominance of her captor.

'Commander, you should keep your crew under better control,' said Uris with the air of a headmaster addressing an unfortunate parent.

Maria instantly shot back her reply. 'If I wasn't wasting my time here all the time, perhaps I could. Not that I would necessarily bother!'

Uris began to speak, but Maria deliberately spoke over the top of him.

'My crew are all adults. They have been confined for eighteen months, and they are entitled to let their hair down.'

'I don't wish to have my guards exposed to the acts of immorality,' said Uris, managing to get his bit in.

As ever Maria countered immediately. 'Then tell your guards to go off somewhere else and leave my crew alone.'

Uris was meeting his match, and he knew it. To be constantly outwitted by this wisp of a female had imposed an unfamiliar burden upon him. He attempted a different tack, first attempting to reactivate his plastic smile.

'Commander, now let's be more cooperative. You must understand that we must take precautions. After all, you come along and invade . . .'

'Invade!' interjected Maria. 'We have come in a craft only fitted for scientific discovery, and you have imprisoned us.'

Uris turned to one of the stooge-like individuals seated next to him who nodded, then spoke. He didn't sound all that intelligent, thought Maria, but Maria welcomed his more forthright style of speech.

'We'd like you to speak to one of your colleagues on the space station,' said the man, who didn't bother to introduce himself.

Maria tried not to show her eagerness at this development. Hopefully it would be Adam, she thought.

Within a few minutes Jack's face appeared on a screen

near where she sat. She noted a camera trained on herself.

'Hello, Maria,' said Jack.

'Hi Jack. It's good to see you. Where's Adam?'

Jack appeared to ignore the question. Instead he replied, 'We're assisting with the technical side of the running of the space station, processing their data and so on. It takes a bit of getting used to . . . We are quite spaced out . . .'

The transmission was suddenly cut short to prevent Jack from saying any more, it seemed. The man next to Uris spoke again.

'You see, commander, your colleagues are happy to cooperate, why not you?'

'You'll have to do better than that,' spat back Maria uncharacteristically and at the same time stood up. 'I have nothing further to say,' she continued. 'I suggest that I be allowed to return to my crew. They're probably on the verge of another naked rampage!'

Uris terminated the meeting by slamming his hand on the table in front of him. He had clearly lost patience and stormed out, leaving the stooges to arrange for Maria's return. Though tempted to needle the other men and guards with whom she came into contact, Maria maintained a steadfast silence which had the effect of enhancing the awe in which she was clearly held. Captive she may be, but prisoner she definitely wasn't.

She was eagerly welcomed by the crew on her return, but first asked to be left alone for a short time with Yvonne to whom she recounted the most recent interrogation and brief conversation with Jack.

'I just can't imagine Jack cooperating,' said Yvonne.

'Neither can I,' replied Maria, 'at least I'm sure he would relish getting into their communications system, perhaps with a view to using it to his advantage.'

Yvonne nodded, then asked, 'What were those last words he said again?'

'It takes a bit of getting used to . . . *We are quite spaced out*,' quoted Maria. 'Do you think there's something strange about that?'

'I don't know,' said Yvonne, sounding serious, 'but you know how cunning Jack is. I wouldn't put it past him to try and give us a message, though it would be a pretty short one.'

'It seems a bit improbable,' said Maria, 'yet I felt that there was something about the way he spoke and . . . it's hard to put into words . . . just the words he used. Jack doesn't use expressions such as "spaced out".'

'No! He doesn't,' said Yvonne, who now appeared to become excited. 'But what could he possibly mean?'

'Let's get Bud,' said Maria. 'He knows Jack better than anyone . . . and Carmel.'

Although fairly large in area, the hut provided little in the way of privacy. However, even though Bud and Carmel's romantic activities had been curtailed, Yvonne found the two secreted in a corner.

'Sorry to interrupt,' announced Yvonne apologetically, 'we need your help.'

The two immediately stood up and followed Yvonne to a different nook where Maria awaited. She divulged her brief conversation with Jack and Bud obliged with an immediate explanation, a broad grin accompanied his reply as well.

'Space language. It's a form of spy communication used in the military. Trust Jack to think of it.'

Maria felt as if she had just won the lottery. 'You mean there was something hidden in what he said?'

'It takes a bit of getting used to. It means it is quite complex,' replied Bud. 'The bit about being spaced out refers to the code itself.'

15

Stephanie melted into the forest at the sight of the children being herded away and the DSP crew being sent back indoors. She wasn't to see either groups for the remainder of the day. With the whole settlement seemingly confined, she embarked upon a mission of wider exploration.

The immediate settlement with which she had become familiar was relatively small. She had gleaned snippets of information from the children's conversations with each other, and knew roughly where to look. She carefully avoided arousing suspicion or drawing attention to herself by asking direct questions. After a long walk down the road which led further inland, she stopped for a rest. She was tired and ravenously hungry. Her energy had been further drained by the practice of intermittently making part of the journey through the forest and thus contending with irregular ground, trees and scrub. Determined to succeed, she set off once more. It was after one of her excursions into the forest, or at least out of it again, that she unexpectedly stumbled across some good fortune in the form of Penny's two friends, Elsa and Mara.

Cautious as ever before exiting the cover of the scrub, Stephanie leapt down an embankment onto the edge of the road. A squeal nearly scared her out of her wits. Sitting — up until Stephanie's arrival peacefully — were the two girls, in the midst of having their lunch. Mara, on realising who it was, yelled in a shrill voice, 'Cecily! You nearly landed on top of us!'

'I'm sorry,' replied Stephanie. 'I didn't know you were there, you were awfully quiet.'

'Mara softened her tone. 'That's all right. We were busy munching. Here, do you want to join us?'

'I haven't anything,' replied Stephanie.

'We've got heaps,' chimed in Elsa, 'you can have as much as you like!'

Stephanie's manners just managed to override the gnawing instinct of the starved wolf within her as she replied, 'Are you sure? I'm not all that hungry!'

Stephanie felt as if she had just uttered the biggest lie that she had ever told. The remark was ignored by the insistent Elsa, who pushed a sandwich into her hand, soon to be followed by a drink in the other. In spite of a desire within her to swallow each sandwich whole, Stephanie nibbled in the fashion of one who has foolishly stated that she isn't hungry.

'You weren't at the clearing this morning,' said Stephanie.

'No,' replied Mara, 'the group of kids who were there were taken away . . . to be asked questions I think . . .'

'What about?' asked Stephanie.

'To see if any of those Earth people told them anything important . . . like they've done to Penny.'

Stephanie's senses bristled at the thought of the children being used unwittingly as spies.

'What has happened to Penny?' asked Stephanie, a note of concern creeping into her voice.

'She got really upset apparently. She doesn't like talking about people behind their backs. That's why Elsa and I haven't been back. We didn't want to end up in the same trouble.'

'What sort of trouble is Penny in?' asked Stephanie.

'Oh, not much herself,' replied Mara. 'Her parents will be the ones to suffer most.'

A cold chill traversed Stephanie's otherwise warm body. She wondered what type of suffering Mara meant. However, she didn't pursue the subject. The three girls finished their lunch and sat chatting idly for another ten minutes. Mara announced that they intended to return home and Stephanie joined them. They led her to quite a large housing estate. In the distance Stephanie thought that she could see what looked like a large air base. She also noticed a few men hovering around the entrance to the estate as they approached. She decided that they were best avoided and quickly made an excuse to turn back.

'Oh!' she exclaimed and stopped in her tracks.

'What's the matter?' asked Mara.

'I must have left it on the ground when we had lunch. I'll have to go back, I'll see you later.'

'Bye then!' said Mara unquestioningly as Stephanie began to move off. She stopped again and turned.

'Which is Penny's house?'

'Sixteen . . . second street on the left,' called back Elsa, 'bye!'

'Bye,' called back Stephanie and quickly moved away, not stopping to look back again.

Recharged by the unexpected lunch, Stephanie decided to reconnoitre the air base that she could see in the distance. She approached it via the forest and eventually drew close enough to see it in more detail. It appeared deserted. The runway areas were huge by comparison with anything with which she was familiar. There were buildings scattered along one side of the perimeter, but no sign of life. She observed the scene for a while, then decided to return to the more familiar territory where her fellow crew members were held. By the time she had begun the return journey it was quite late and the sun was already setting. The moon had been rising earlier and earlier, and gave the prospect of some darkness later in the evening.

Later that night no one in the hut which held the DSP crew was aware of a small figure approaching through the forest. She crept forward to the tree that she had indicated to Carmel and Loretta and hoped that they had managed to deposit her supplies. She was ignorant of the lengths to which her colleagues had gone to fulfill their objective. Whilst Gerda and Paul had so blatantly distracted the guards, Carmel had leapt into the forest, ostensibly to retrieve her slacks which had been expertly flung by Bud, so that they had landed near the predetermined drop point. As she bent to retrieve the slacks, Carmel quickly effected another manouevre. Under her T-shirt she wore the halter which normally harnessed Gerda's above average bosoms. Though moderately endowed herself, Carmel was no match for the voluptuous Gerda, this anatomical fact leaving an abundance of space within the oversized brassière for two moderate-sized packages, which had been moulded, more or less, into spherical shapes and distended the fabric containing them even more than the usual incumbent objects.

As Carmel bent, she shoe-horned out the packages, grasped her slacks and ran back to the hut. Many hours later Stephanie searched for what she expected to be a single parcel. On coming across a spherical object, she grasped it and studied it, appearing slightly puzzled. The second package was nearby and soon spotted as well. Stephanie wondered why Carmel had bothered to make two rather than one, though she later concluded, incorrectly, that the reason must have been to separate food from toiletries. Carmel had taken the opportunity to divide the goods this way, but only as an afterthought.

Stephanie shrunk back into the forest, grasping her treasure. Hunger had long overtaken her again. It had been a long time since the unexpected lunch. She wondered how she would have survived without it, and shuddered at the thought. Her target was a spot near a stream which she had selected earlier, and to which she had moved her belongings. It was now dark as the moon had crossed the night sky at last and Stephanie felt much safer. The babbling of the stream became her compass in the gloom and she sighed with relief when she eventually dropped onto a flat piece of ground at her new-found base. She began to open the first package like a child opening a present.

'Mmm ... food,' she uttered aloud. She decided, contrary to her upbringing, that on this occasion eating took precedence over cleanliness, though she wisely conserved some of the menu for the next morning.

She then attacked the other parcel, half guessing, half hoping, about its contents. She recognised a basic pack that each member of the shuttle crew would have brought down from the DSP. It consisted of soap, hair shampoo and a few first aid items. She presumed that Carmel had donated her entire pack; no doubt Loretta or one of the others would share theirs in return. Added to the standard issue was a clean pair of knickers, which she recognised as Carmel's, the latter assuming that under current circumstances, Stephanie wouldn't be fussy about sharing.

Stephanie laid out the contents of the second parcel, then slipped her dress over her head. She then removed a tight band of material which she had tied around her chest to flatten the glands which she paradoxically had been trying to display as larger for the last eighteen months. She sighed with relief and carefully patted the bruised organs. Her knickers were then slid off and dropped straight into a nearby pool. Within seconds she had waded into the stream and had nestled her bottom onto the rocks at the base. The water was cool, but the air was warm, which proved a perfect combination. Having shampooed the tangled hair, washed herself all over at least three times and apologised to the fish for the pollution she had caused, she lay back and for the first time thought well of this strange planet. Finally she stepped from the water and sat on a small towel which had encircled the toiletries and allowed her body to dry naturally in the warm air. The tunic, after receiving a thorough beating, became a thin mattress on which to slip into a deep and satisfying slumber.

* * *

'How does this space code work?' asked Yvonne sounding intrigued.

'It's based on the old Morse code system,' replied Bud, 'except that you use short spaces instead of dots and long spaces instead of dashes.'

'But how are the spaces used?' said Yvonne.

'You can use different spacing between words or lines or paragraphs, anything you like, or the gaps after the words at the end of each line; it depends on the length of your message and the amount of text that you have available.'

'I've never heard of it,' exclaimed Maria.

'It didn't have much practical use,' continued Bud. 'Once you know it's being used, it's relatively easy to crack.'

'Do many people know about it?'

'All the techs do,' replied Carmel, 'Jack taught us early in the mission, when there wasn't much to do. We used to send cryptic messages to each other.'

'It's a brilliant idea,' said Yvonne. 'I don't see how we can use it, though, we don't have access to a computer.'

Carmel astounded them with her next statement. 'Actually we do!'

Her dumbfounded colleagues stared at her, Maria thinking that she should never be surprised at what Carmel may have up her sleeve. She asked the obvious question.

'OK Carmel spill the beans, where's the computer? Under the floorboards?'

'No, but there's someone who can use theirs . . . or ours in the shuttle.'

Carmel continued as her audience hung on every word.

'Did you notice that messy looking kid that Loretta and I were speaking to?'

The others nodded.

'Well . . . that kid was Stephanie in disguise!'

Maria and Bud gasped. Yvonne threw her head back and laughed. She was the first to speak.

'Life will be very boring one day . . .'

'I don't believe it,' interrupted Maria, 'it's impossible!'

Carmel smiled, then related the facts surrounding Stephanie's masterful deception.

'Is that what you wanted to speak to me about?' asked Maria at the conclusion.

'Yes,' replied Carmel. 'I'm sorry we didn't tell you the day before . . . I was afraid that they might torture you or something.'

'Why is everyone so worried about me being tortured?' said Maria, glancing at Yvonne. 'So what was the purpose of the striptease?'

'To drop off some supplies to Stephanie. I borrowed Gerda's bra and hid a couple of packages in it. I dropped them when I retrieved my slacks.

'Very clever!' said Maria. 'You can bet that Gerda had the guards' complete attention!'

'We figured as much,' said Carmel with a grin. 'Actually it was Loretta's idea. She even tried to talk Gerda into having Paul pull down her pants, but she was a bit reluctant to go that far, especially as we wouldn't tell her exactly what we were doing.'

'I think that she went quite far enough!' remarked Maria. 'Now . . . how do we use all of this to our advantage?'

A long discussion ensued. It was eventually interrupted by the arrival of the evening meal and then it resumed and continued well into the night, much of the time being spent teaching Maria and Yvonne the finer points of the code. The following morning, Maria approached Uris and his colleagues in a negotiating mood.

'I wish to make a deal,' she announced bluntly.

Uris responded with a suspicious stare, then spoke defensively. 'What sort of deal?'

'I insist on more freedom for my crew. After all, they aren't about to sprout wings and fly away. In return I will provide you with some information, though I need to communicate with my colleagues on your space station and I also demand assurances regarding their safety.'

Uris applied his plastic smile and replied, 'Your attitude is improving, Commander. However, you are in no position to give orders . . .'

'Take it or leave it,' interrupted Maria sharply.

Uris rested back in his chair. He seemed more relaxed than the day before.

'I think we can come to an arrangement, Commander.'

Within half an hour Uris and Maria had thrashed out an agreement. One of Maria's concessions was that she would type instructions to Jack on the space station, this being the perfect arrangement for the transmission of hidden messages. Ironically, Uris had been mistakenly suspicious of verbal communications and had played directly into Maria's hands. The limiting factor in Maria's case, however, was that any replies from Jack would need time and study for analysis, and Maria did not have the means of retaining any information. Nevertheless, all transmissions, it was hoped, would be kept in the communications centre, the plan being for Stephanie to somehow break in after hours, as she had done before.

To use Stephanie meant gaining access to her, there being a limit to the subterfuge which had been used when Gerda acted as a decoy. Maria fought hard for the easing of restrictions on her crew, but she only managed to win a rather inadequate compromise.

'You will instruct us on the use of your shuttle, and I can promise you all the freedom you wish,' said Uris with the air of victory in his voice.

Maria knew only too well that the major reason for their confinement was to keep them away from the shuttle; telling Uris how to operate it would result in its immediate disappearance. It was a no win situation. She refused to concede this point and returned to her colleagues, somewhat grim-faced.

'It looks like one way signals only for the time being,' she said as she recounted her dealings to Yvonne and Bud.

'Number one priority, then, should be to let them know upstairs that Stephanie has escaped undetected. I've been thinking that they might accidentally blow the whistle, thinking that Stephanie's been kidnapped or something,' said Bud.

'You're right,' replied Maria immediately. 'Let's get to work then. I'm due to return and start transmitting this afternoon.'

'What's the story on the rest of us being allowed out?' asked Yvonne.

'Something's happened. I don't know what. I suspect that they think that we may have influenced someone amongst the children or turned one of them into a spy or something.'

'Which is true!' remarked Bud.

Maria shook her head. 'If you mean Stephanie, no, I don't think so, it's someone else. Anyway, we can go out, but we are to stay away from the edge of the clearing, and there is no contact allowed with anyone.'

That afternoon Maria returned and issued her first text. She was supervised closely, but her instructions to Jack were very simple and could in no way be construed as containing any hidden messages. Little did her invigilators know that the pattern of Maria's typing sent a clear message regarding Stephanie's brilliant escape and the fact that, for the time being, she would be unable to interpret any response.

The nature of Maria's transmissions was trivial to say the least. They implied that Jack required certain signals in order to release any information. Maria also agreed initially only to provide basic technical information about life support systems and basic internal operations of the DSP. Nevertheless it seemed to satisfy the captors, especially the scale of technology which was used.

On the space station, Jack suppressed a smile as he realised immediately that Maria was using his code. He was expert enough to interpret it as he read the largely irrelevant main text. It required exceptional powers of self-control on his behalf, however, to maintain a straight face as he digested the fact that Stephanie was on the loose and her very existence not even suspected by their captors. At the end of his written 'conversation' with Maria, he casually made a demand.

'Er . . . there's a couple of things that I don't understand . . . I'll need some help from our captain.'

Saying nothing in reply, one of the supervisors left. After about twenty minutes he returned with Adam and issued an instruction.

'You may only discuss the transmission . . . nothing else.'

This was the first time that Adam had come into contact with any member of the DSP crew, apart from Alex, since their capture. Jack's affable smile proved a great tonic to Adam. What he was about to see, however, would make him euphoric.

'There's some gaps in this transmission, Captain,' said Jack benignly, 'I need you to fill in the spaces.'

Adam knew immediately what was meant by Jack's crafty language and in perusing the text, he literally read between the lines. He also possessed Jack's ability to interpret the code on sight. His eyes widened at the sight of the hidden revelation, and he suppressed his excitement with great difficulty. Then he indulged in irrelevant banter about fictitious details relating to the main text. Within minutes he would be back with Alex and sharing the secret, as was Jack with the remainder of his technicians imprisoned on the space station. Though it seemed an impossible task for Stephanie to somehow free them all, it gave them a ray of hope. It was now up to them to create a situation whereby they could use their young colleague's freedom to their advantage.

Earlier, Stephanie had awoken to the joy of feeling clean and well rested. This inspired a fresh enthusiasm which would unfortunately be dashed as the restricted access to her colleagues became apparent. She had approached the clearing and noted the absence of children. She then managed to signal Carmel from the cover of the forest, but Carmel had clearly gestured for her to stay away. As a result of this and the prospect of going hungry loomed again, she decided to track down Penny and take the risk of infiltrating the local community.

After the long walk to the other settlement, she approached the entrance cautiously, especially as she would have to run the gauntlet of the guards. However, as she was a master of deception, the guards were easily bemused, but only after a false start.

'What are you doing out, Miss?' questioned one of them.

'I went out early,' replied Stephanie.

'Let's have your card,' he continued, stern-faced.

Stephanie assumed that he meant the ID card and

handed it across. He stared at it, then looked back at her.

'You're not supposed to be out,' he stated.

Stephanie just shrugged and replied, 'I didn't go far . . . I dropped something yesterday and went back to get it.'

The guard frowned. He appeared suspicious. He fingered Stephanie's card, then announced as he flashed it in front of her face, 'I'm going to check up on this.'

With that he entered a small box-like hut near the gate, Stephanie could just make out a computer terminal inside, at which the guard tapped away. She hoped that her forged card would stand up to his scrutiny. He returned soon after, slapping the card on his hand. Stephanie studied him closely, summoning her considerable powers of analysis; she possessed a sixth sense when it came to deciphering an individual's external expressions. The guard squinted as if he were about to interrogate her, yet his mouth was relaxed, unlike that of a person who had discovered anything significant. So before he spoke, Stephanie knew that her ID had passed the test, but from his eyes she knew that she was still in for a hard time. She would be ready.

'Your card doesn't match!' the guard exclaimed.

'Match what? The colour of the sky!' replied Stephanie, sounding quite insolent.

The guard was taken aback by this unexpected display of defiance. It was clear that he had not anticipated having to formulate his next question so soon and lost the advantage in the exchange by stuttering, 'It-t . . . it doesn't match your age . . . you're supposed to be nearly sixteen.'

Stephanie was inwardly amused at how accurate this statement was in relation to her true age. She demolished the guard with a reply which belied her true nature.

'So I am. What do I have to do? Show you my tits!'

Both guards appeared genuinely shocked at Stephanie's verbal display of vulgarity, but it certainly had the desired effect, in that it effectively torpedoed any further attempts by the guard to exert his authority.

'Don't be disgusting,' he said and threw the card back at Stephanie, who caught it deftly and stalked away.

She soon located Penny's house. Like most of the others it was a bland box-like structure, though it had a small garden with flowers that immediately attracted Stephanie's interest. She approached the garden and studied the display. Some varieties she recognised; others were totally unfamiliar and had an exotic tropical appearance. Nearby, the door of the house had opened silently and a tall figure observed Stephanie, who had been distracted by the beauty of the garden.

'You like the flowers?'

Stephanie spun immediately and observed a tall, sandy-haired young man. He wore a faint smile, which gave his expression a kindly appearance. He was indisputably related to Penny.

'They're beautiful!' replied Stephanie. Her lips could have quite easily uttered: '. . . and so are you!' However, instead she remained silent and waited for the young man to speak again. He didn't and it was Stephanie who eventually activated the conversation.

'I came to see Penny.'

'Come inside,' replied the young man.

Stephanie obliged without hesitation and was led into a neat but simply furnished sitting room. The youth offered her a seat and introduced himself.

'I'm Leonard, Penny's brother.'

'I'm Cecily,' replied Stephanie. 'Isn't Penny at home?'

Leonard shook his head. He stared intently at Stephanie as if to assess her reliability. She could tell that something troubled him.

'No.' he replied.

'Is she all right?' asked Stephanie before he could continue.

Leonard sighed. 'I suppose so. How well do you know her? Are you a good friend?'

Stephanie sensed that Penny was indeed in some sort of trouble and probed further without giving a direct answer to the question.

'I like Penny a lot and I want to help her if I can. You can trust me.'

'You can't trust anyone around here,' sneered Leonard. 'You should be careful making statements like that.'

'I'm new,' said Stephanie, 'I don't know anything about this place.'

'Where are you from?' asked Leonard.

'A long way away,' replied Stephanie truthfully.

Leonard stared at Stephanie. Obviously neither party was willing to give anything away. The silence was broken by the sound of a whistle in the distance. Leonard shot out of his chair as if someone had released a spring under his bottom. He rushed to the window and exclaimed, 'They're looking for someone!'

Stephanie flashed to his side as a strange premonition swept her mind. It was confirmed as she recognised the guard with whom she had the altercation. There appeared to be men stationing themselves at either end of the street and others going door to door. Stephanie astounded Leonard by suddenly snapping an order. 'Your mother, where's her room?'

Leonard appeared dumbfounded and unable to reply.

'Are you going to help me or not?' she demanded.

'Yes, but . . .'

'No buts. Now where is her room? Quickly!'

'Come, I'll show you,' replied the bewildered Leonard.

Stephanie elbowed her way past him as he led her to the rear of the house.

'I'm sorry about this,' she stated as she began to rummage in some drawers. She pulled her tunic over her head. Leonard, feeling embarrassed, started to leave, but Stephanie restrained him.

'Don't go too far away. I might need you!'

'Very well, I just thought . . .'

'Does your mother have any make-up?' interrupted Stephanie.

'No . . . at least I don't think so . . .'

'Go outside and get me some dirt,' interrupted Stephanie again. 'Just a bit . . . Try not to look too obvious and don't catch anyone's eye.'

Leonard obeyed his juvenile commander, though he wasn't sure why. Such was the force of Stephanie's personality that it just seemed to be the correct thing to do. When he returned Stephanie was sitting topless in front of a small mirror and hastily tying up her hair.

'And some water,' she said, without turning, as Leonard entered with the strange offering, He turned and left in order to comply with the latest demand. When he returned, Stephanie was wearing one of his mother's brassières and was in the process of stuffing it with various items of clothing.

'Thanks,' she remarked as Leonard returned with the strange items that she had requested. She immediately made a paste out of the dirt and water. In anticipation Leonard left to obtain a towel. When he returned he watched as Stephanie carefully blended the clay-coloured mud around her eyes, then drew her fingernails delicately through the area. The nett result was a myriad of fine crows feet near the corner of each eye. She then carefully applied the mixture under the eyes, giving the impression of the dark rings that those who have burnt the midnight oil find themselves familiar with the next morning. Some apparent 'sun spots' completed the ageing process. The face completed, Stephanie leapt up and further embarrassed her co-conspirator. 'Pull my knickers away from my bum and stuff these things down . . .'

Leonard approached gingerly and handed Stephanie the towel. She smiled, thus breaking the tension, and began to wipe her hands and then continued her directions. 'Go on . . . stuff them really tight!'

Her hands cleaned, she took over the task herself, much to Leonard's relief. She moulded the wadding into a rotund shape, then pulled a scarf up tightly through her crutch to indent the stuffing into an artificial natal cleft.

Five minutes later the door to door investigators arrived to be greeted by the large posterior of a woman who was stooped over and apparently absorbed in her gardening. Her hair was concealed under a tight scarf and she only rose to an upright position after being challenged on the second occasion. As she turned and faced the two men who had entered the property, she drew her dirty hand across her face leaving a brown smudge on her cheek.

'We're looking for a kid . . . about thirteen or fourteen . . . dark hair . . . have you seen her?' questioned one of the men.

The woman shook her head and muttered softly, 'No!'

'We have to search the house,' continued the man.

'Go ahead,' replied the woman and immediately turned her attention back to the garden.

Between the time Stephanie had completed her disguise and the time of arrival of the investigators, Leonard had tidied his mother's room and placed Stephanie's clothes amongst Penny's. The men entered the house to be greeted by Leonard, who was casually seated and apparently reading a book.

'What's up?' he asked.

'We're looking for a kid. Sorry, we have to search every house, we won't mess anything up . . .'

Leonard shrugged and returned to his reading. The box-like houses were easy to search and the men had soon completed their task.

'Thanks,' said one of them as they trooped past Leonard again. They quickly moved on to the next dwelling, ignoring the gardener, who was still bent over the flower patch.

Stephanie waited until the men were well down the street and then waddled inside. She immediately flopped into a seat and looked across at Leonard. A big smile appeared on her face as she spoke.

'Thanks a million . . .'

'I take it that you're the runaway kid that they were looking for,' said Leonard. 'Mind filling me in?'

Stephanie nodded as she considered to what extent she should 'fill in' the person who unquestioningly had just saved her from certain capture.

'I'm trying to help the Earth people . . . the ones who are captured.'

'You are? Then you know that we are attempting to do the same!'

'Let me get out of this get up first,' said Stephanie. 'Then we can talk properly.'

She disappeared into the back room again and removed the disguise. She suddenly felt acutely embarrassed that she had appeared naked before Leonard, though at the time, in the urgency of the situation, it hadn't even crossed her mind. Before long she had rejoined him and sat child-like, swinging her legs. Leonard obviously found some difficulty fathoming the complex individual in front of him; the transformation had been spectacular in the extreme.

'That's better,' sighed Stephanie, shaking her hair off her face, 'I'm sorry about the dress up party. I had to think quickly!'

'You were brilliant,' replied Leonard, 'You're obviously an expert at this sort of thing.'

Stephanie smiled and changed the subject. 'Do you know

what they plan to do with the Earth people?'

'Well, they certainly plan to keep them, and use them. My father . . . he's a scientist, and some of his colleagues, were trying to arrange their release. They think that they should be welcomed, not imprisoned. It is a great opportunity to share knowledge. Unfortunately the administration thinks otherwise. They want to treat them the same as all other new arrivals from Earth.'

Stephanie hung on every word. She was to discover, as Maria had, the nature and history of the Earth colony, but Leonard was also to reveal that control had very much fallen into the wrong hands and that those in power had designs on the planet itself. The nuclear fuel and associated technology on the DSP had been earmarked by this gang of thugs and was in danger of tipping the scales in the direction of evil. The innocent Penny had been caught up in the counter movement by way of her father voicing his dissent, especially after she had been spotted conversing with the DSP crew members.

Having divulged his information, Leonard requested some compensation. 'So . . . what's your story?'

'I can't tell you much . . . I . . .'

A timely interruption arrived in the form of Penny and her mother, the latter being an attractive tall woman, though dark-haired in contrast to her fair children. She bore no resemblance whatsoever to the bulky, buxom figure that Stephanie had portrayed in her earlier ruse.

'Cecily!' exclaimed Penny. 'What are you doing here?'

Penny's mother appeared confused and frightened, thought Stephanie. Before she could answer, Leonard immediately recounted every detail of the events which had occurred since Stephanie's arrival. At the conclusion, all three members of the family turned to Stephanie, who bit her lip and responded carefully.

'I'm afraid that you will have to trust me. I can't tell

you everything.'

Penny stared excitedly at this mysterious figure who had suddenly injected excitement into her normally mundane existence.

'Can't you tell us anything else?' she asked desperately.

'Perhaps I could speak to your father,' said Stephanie, eager to deflect the requests for further personal details.

'I'm afraid that's impossible,' replied Penny's mother. 'He's been detained.' She bowed her head as she spoke and Stephanie noticed that both Leonard and Penny produced expressions of concern, if not alarm. Stephanie herself suddenly began to feel the weight of responsibility on her young shoulders as the predicament appeared to be growing rapidly more complex. However, being only sixteen, a more pressing need suddenly engulfed her.

'I'm starved,' she stated.

Penny's mother leapt up, happy to find something to distract her from her melancholia.

'You poor thing,' she said in a motherly manner. 'Here, Penny, come and help.'

Stephanie rose to assist but was politely told to relax. She found herself alone again with Leonard.

'How old are you, Cecily?' he asked.

'That depends,' she answered with a cheeky smile.

'You don't give anything away do you?'

'No, but I promise to tell you everything at some stage,' said Stephanie more sincerely. 'How old are you?'

'I have no secrets. I'm twenty-two,' replied Leonard with a laugh.

'What do you do?' asked Stephanie.

'I'm an engineer. I don't suppose you know much about that sort of thing.'

'I know a bit,' said Stephanie, the cheeky expression returning. For some reason she felt uncomfortable and she couldn't figure why. She normally had no problems relating to males, at least not the ones with whom she was familiar. This male was different, though. She was attracted to him; she even found herself wanting to sit next to him and touch him. It made her feel embarrassed and uncomfortable. Penny and her mother rescued her from her feelings.

'Here, Cecily,' said the mother, 'have as much as you like.'

'Thank you, Mrs . . . I'm sorry . . . I don't even know your last name!'

'Hutchinson,' said Leonard as he also eyed off the delicacies and was promptly warned to take his turn.

Her body refuelled, Stephanie turned her thoughts back to more important matters.

'I'll have to find some way of getting back to the forest . . .'

'Do you have to go?' asked Penny.

'Yes. Besides, I'm putting you in danger being here . . . What's the best way out?'

'I'll get you out,' announced Leonard, 'I have to drive out later.'

Leonard left and returned with a sort of truck which he parked close to the front door. He loaded a few odds and ends and a sack-like structure which contained Stephanie hidden inside. She felt herself being driven off. The vehicle stopped at one stage and she heard voices. It then continued its journey and eventually came to a halt again. Stephanie found herself being lifted out and, on removing her covering, found herself at the edge of the forest.

She stood close to Leonard and looked up at him. Her heart pounded. An individual whose feelings were normally under total control, she felt acutely uncomfortable. Not knowing what to say, she suddenly encircled his neck with her arms and kissed him firmly. Then she ran off into the forest, not even turning to say goodbye.

Leonard watched the strange, secretive girl disappear

from sight. Was she a child or a woman? The impulsive kiss provided no clue, though a more astute individual might have recognised the awakenings of passion and romance in that kiss. Nevertheless, it left an impression on the young man and he would continue to think about it. Stephanie too would think about it, though she would battle with her feelings and try to dismiss them. She hurried back to her hideaway in the forest and waited until the few hours of darkness between moonlight and dawn. She tried to rest, but her mind was filled with the day's activities and her fixation with Leonard. Her mind even drifted off into fantasising about their meeting. She imagined him coming up behind her when she had been virtually naked and embracing her . . . and the kiss . . . The more she thought about it, the more erotic the memory of the other events became, especially when he had exposed her buttocks at her request.

Though far from her mind at the time, embarrassment and eroticism intertwined in her thoughts and she even imagined him delving further as he placed his hand between her knickers and her exposed rump. She banished the intrusive erotic thoughts from her mind by removing her clothes and plunging into the cold stream. The shock of the cold water reset her priorities and she laid her plans in detail for the night.

The moon eventually completed its passage and Stephanie set off in the direction of the shuttle. She found that the guard around the clearing where the DSP crew was billeted had been lifted, but in turn used for the shuttle instead. Her plans altered, she set off for the clearing and approached through the forest as usual. She froze as her keen senses perceived a sound ahead, an unfamiliar sound. Having driven her own erotic thoughts from her mind she was soon to have them reactivated in a different form. Edging her way forward, she made out human forms in the small clearing ahead. The muffled sounds were unfamiliar and she continued her forward approach, the sounds becoming more intense as she did so. Eventually she obtained a clear view. Gerda and Paul, she mouthed as she came to witness the act of human lovemaking. She stared in wonderment, having always imagined the act to be slow and romantic in nature. She was amazed, if not horrified as she watched what she regarded as the most delicate area of the female body assaulted frenetically and with the apparent power of a jack hammer. Paradoxically, Gerda appeared to submit totally to the piston-like assault. With legs opened like gates, her breasts swung wildly with each collision and she uttered stifled, though unmistakably euphoric cries of ecstacy.

For once in her short life Stephanie was clearly at a loss as to what to do. To gain access to her colleagues was a dream come true, but to sidle up to individuals so engaged and tap them on the shoulder must surely be poor form. Apart from that she felt extremely uncomfortable and embarrassed, as if she were snooping. However, with so much at stake she dallied. Hopefully they would finish, and when they were dressed she could pretend to suddenly come upon the scene. Unfortunately, having gained the opportunity to indulge their passions in what they had assumed was seclusion, Gerda and Paul were in no mind to bring their erotic proceedings prematurely to an end.

Stephanie's sex education continued unabated and in expanded detail as the two lovers explored the permutations of locking their pelves from different directions and in unimaginable positions. Stephanie's mind momentarily wandered as she recalled her earlier erotic thoughts. They seemed trivial compared with the true life performance which she now witnessed and she wondered if she could ever successfully submit herself to such imaginative invasion. But she became mesmerised by the sight of the raw power of Paul's buttocks, the frenzied contractions driving him deep into his companion. She suddenly felt flushed. A surging feeling traversed her own pelvis and she developed an uncontrollable desire to be penetrated herself with the same power. She even found herself toying with the idea that she would submit herself to Paul and beg him to serve her need . . . though after Gerda was fully satisfied. She gave a slight giggle at the unlikely thought, though the aching desire refused to subside.

Nubile and ripe as the young virgin was, common sense prevailed as she bludgeoned the more pressing needs of the safety of her crew members into her mind. Sex would have to wait . . . unfortunately! She concluded that her two colleagues may well continue their exercises for hours and with a smirk on her face and a dull ache clawing at her aroused but unsatisfied organs, she inched her way around the clearing. As she drew away, she barely heard the lovers' convulsive cries of climactic ecstasy. She had already set her sights on the communication centre, and her friends' copulatory activities would soon be dismissed from her mind.

There were guards strategically placed to watch the wider area near the clearing where the DSP members were held, but fortunately the communciations centre, as on previous occasions, stood unwatched. On her previous visits, Stephanie had been preoccupied with pilfering data and transporting it to the shuttle. In fact her original plan had been to sneak into the shuttle and review the stolen information. Now she would study it at its source and expand her knowledge of this odd community.

16

High above the planet a transmission was received by the external communications centre on the space station . . . or was it received? A call sign lit up, but nothing seemed to follow. A message was flashed to the command centre and an immediate instruction issued to check the DSP prisoners, none of whom were in an operational area. Anderson was summoned and, having been woken from sleep, entered the command centre in a positively surly mood.

The signal was retrieved and replayed, but it provided no useful information. Anderson was suspicious, if not paranoid, and ordered the DSP members to be brought before him. For the first time since capture Adam had the satisfaction of seeing his colleagues, at least those on the station, to be in good spirits.

Anderson had already summoned his counterpart on the surface of the planet, the unfortunate individual being unable to offer any explanation. Furthermore, for some reason, his equipment was unable to locate the source of the dummy transmission. As Adam and his group stood before Anderson, the remaining crew on the surface were being paraded outside the hut and the latter searched. Daylight was just breaking and some had already been awake. Others, two in particular, had been aroused from a deep sleep and stood somewhat bleary-eyed.

'I want to know what you know about this?' demanded Anderson as he played the transmission to the audience. Adam shrugged and replied on behalf of his crew.

'Someone commenced a transmission, then stopped . . . What do you expect us to know about it?'

Anderson was lost for words, but Jack and Helen were not lost for a thought, and the thought consisted of one word . . . Stephanie.

Their eyes scanned the call sign, its configuration, its punctuation and the barely susceptible dots which followed. Their hearts pounded as they realised that the space station's computer had been infected with a virus . . . but to what purpose and when would it strike?

After a futile display of histrionics, the two separate groups of DSP members were allowed to return to their respective quarters, those on the ground being somewhat bewildered, but those aloft buzzed with anticipation.

As the sun rose Stephanie sat in the middle of the stream, attempting to revitalise herself after a long night's work bent over a computer terminal in the local communications building. She had discovered disturbing news indeed, especially in relation to sinister plans for the DSP and its members. It was time to act, quickly and decisively. She gathered her thoughts and tried to dispel feelings of nervousness as she contemplated putting them into action. If only she had help!

When she had stowed away on the shuttle, Stephanie and her colleagues who were to remain on board the DSP wore their usual 'cat suits' in contrast to those who were 'Earth'-bound. Stephanie now retrieved the suit and some other items which she had hastily grabbed to bring with her. She then set to work on her hair, her make-up and her body. If she was going to wage war, she was going to do it in style. The make-up was applied to theatrical standards, accentuating a naturally attractive face. The tailored fluid-filled bags, which normally augmented her bust line, were placed in position for the first time since landing and then the figure-hugging suit pulled up, being unzipped strategically in front. Stephanie had lost in the region of four kilograms in weight since landing, which only added to the litheness of her figure. Finally she donned her belt and tucked two line guns in each side, having grabbed them as she left the DSP.

The impressive looking adventure woman now headed for the shuttle. She had planned to bale up the guards and lock them in the hut, but as luck would have it, there were none there. They had in fact been ordered back to the clearing to form an intensive ring around the hut. Stephanie ran to the shuttle and climbed aboard. She seized upon the flight computer and commenced programming a full take off and docking procedure with the DSP. She set the times and coordinates on automatic, then concealed the whole entry with a security code so that it could not be altered. She prayed that the remainder of her plans would work out; otherwise an empty shuttle would be making its way home to base.

Would the remainder of the operation proceed so smoothly? Only time would tell, she thought, as she cut through the forest and approached the housing settlement at which she had spent the previous day. She checked the time before leaving the forest and determined that she should wait fifteen minutes. Though glad for the rest, her anxiety grew as she tried to formulate the rest of the plan.

'Now!' she exclaimed at the appropriate time and scurried towards the guard post of the housing estate. The guards bothered little to watch the approach to their gate; not that Stephanie used the approach anyway. She was on them before they knew it and found themselves staring down the barrel of a gun. The line guns, though not designed to inflict grievous bodily harm, looked formidable to anyone who didn't know their true purpose as they had extended barrels plus sights.

'Freeze!' yelled Stephanie as she pointed the menacing weapon at her adversaries.

The two guards, who happened to be the same as the ones who had challenged Stephanie the day before, cowered at the sight of the gun. They stared wide-eyed at the apparition, not for one second associating the dominating female with the insolent child who had challenged them in a different manner the day before.

'Wh . . . who are you?' stammered one of them, who appeared to be in fear of his life.

'Your executioner if you don't do as you are told!' spat Stephanie in a most convincing manner. 'Now . . . inside . . . Against the wall . . . and hands on your head!' she commanded. She then added in a vicious tone which belied her beauty, 'If you animals dare try anything I'll kill you . . . and I mean it!'

The men were truly convinced and had no mind to argue. To their further amazement, Stephanie proceeded to access their computer and had Uris on the screen, minus his plastic grin, which had been replaced by an expression of complete bewilderment. Stephanie once again didn't mince words.

'Your communications will shortly be taken over, as will those of your space station. You are to follow my instructions, and I warn you to comply.'

'What do you want?' asked Uris nervously.

Stephanie attempted an evil laugh . . . with moderate effect. 'I want your head . . . I've been sent to stop you . . . for good! Now . . . you have a man called Hutchinson in custody. I want him brought to this gate . . . and I want the Earth people released and returned to their shuttle and allowed to board without interference.'

Uris seemed too stunned to answer.

'Do it now . . .' shouted Stephanie and flicked off the computer. She then concurrently tantalised and terrorised her detainees by resting one cheek of her buttocks on the desk and drawing up the corresponding knee, allowing the other leg to fall to the floor and arched her back, thrusting her ample bust forward. At the same time she menacingly waved the gun at the two men and elevated their tension to fever pitch by not making a sound, but subjecting them to a penetrating stare.

Within minutes a vehicle arrived with two men. One, with fair hair, was unmistakenly a clone of Penny and Leonard; the other was quickly ordered against the wall with the two guards.

'Secure them, Mr Hutchinson,' ordered Stephanie as she reached down her cleavage and produced the necessary equipment. Penny's father did as he was asked. He appeared wide-eyed and puzzled but didn't dare question. The men secured, Stephanie reactivated the computer and had the now morbid Uris in front of her again.

'Say goodbye to your communications . . . I suggest that you surrender and cause no further trouble to this planet.'

Stephanie then typed in a command and the screen went blank . . . as did the whole communcations network.

'Come with me!' she exclaimed to Penny's father and led him quickly to the vehicle. 'Take me to your house.'

'Who are you?' he asked.

Stephanie smiled, her character completely changing, much to the amazement of her driver.

'I'll explain when we get there . . . Hurry!'

The journey only took minutes and they both tumbled out of the vehicle and ran up the steps of the small dwelling. Penny had already flung the door open and screamed, 'Dad! It's Dad. Who is . . .?'

'This woman has just rescued me!' interrupted Mr Hutchinson. By this time Mrs Hutchinson and Leonard had also appeared and rushed to embrace their loved one, but with one eye drawn to his glamorous associate. Leonard penetrated Stephanie with his eyes and he gasped, 'You're Cecily. My God . . . what next!'

Penny and her mother froze, open-mouthed as they grasped the identity of this individual of multiple appearances.

'Actually my name is Stephanie,' said the now grinning figure before them. Penny stared in girlish wonderment at the individual who, up until now, had been a child like herself. Stephanie noticed Penny's bewilderment and took her by the hand. Penny muttered softly, almost apologetically, 'Where are you from?'

'I'm from another planet, honey, and today I must return . . . but I'll never forget you. I had to come and say goodbye.'

She then turned to Leonard, who looked equally dumbfounded. Could this embodiment of perfect womanhood be the impulsive child who had kissed him the day before? Or for that matter the ridiculous individual in the garden with all the padding on her bottom! Once again not knowing what to say to Leonard, Stephanie approached him, embraced him and kissed him. It was not the kiss of the impulsive girl of the day before, but a prolonged, passionate, even erotic kiss, enhanced by the embrace in which she pressed herself close to him, down the full length of her body, pushing her knee between his legs and gripping one of his legs with her thighs.

Reluctantly, Stephanie broke from the embrace and sounded an urgent tone. 'We must go. I've knocked out all communications, but it won't last forever. Mr Hutchinson, I know that you have colleagues ready to take over. This is your chance, but if you can drive me to the clearing where my colleagues were held first.'

'Yes, of course,' replied Mr Hutchinson and they both

leapt back into the vehicle. As they drew away Stephanie's eyes flicked back and forth between Penny and Leonard. Would she ever see them again? she wondered. Their minds thought the same.

Back at the clearing, Stephanie soon found her colleagues gone and the area deserted. She hastened to the communications centre, activated the computer terminal and typed in a security code and prepared for a confrontation. She had formed a mental picture of Anderson from what she could glean from her hours of analysis of the records the night before. She was to find that he was not the jellyfish that Uris was and that a hard battle was to be fought, especially as she was female.

Stephanie demanded to speak to Adam, once again not revealing her identity and lacing her dialogue with threats. Anderson responded with a stonewall intransigence which ate up valuable time and also allowed those on the surface to commence tracing her whereabouts. She stuck grimly to her verbal assault and noted the time carefully, then issued an ultimatum.

'In ten seconds, Commander, your whole space station will be paralysed. It might even fall out of the sky. Don't say that I didn't warn you!'

Anderson went to reply, but Stephanie counted over the top of him, eventually approaching zero: 'Three . . . two . . . one!'

Anderson remained pig-headed to the last, but on completing her count, the space station lit up with major malfunctions in virtually every system. It was not as Stephanie planned; she had hoped to secure the release of her colleagues first, but she had no way of stopping the virus that she had injected the night before. Hopefully Jack would have recognised her efforts and would be able to turn it to his advantage, especially in the chaos which must surely have erupted on the station.

Time was now precious. She only had minutes to reach the shuttle before it too automatically responded to her preprogrammed commands and there was no way of stopping it. The crew in fact was already on board and had ascertained this fact and the time of departure and that Stephanie was still missing. Showing that they weren't lacking in resourcefullness, the DSP crew had imprisoned the guards in the hut near the runway. Maria, Yvonne and Bud were in the forward area of the shuttle and Carmel craned her neck over their shoulders in anticipation of Stephanie's arrival.

Stephanie was aware of a sound in the distance to her rear but concentrated on running towards the shuttle. Eventually she reached the end of the road and ran the last few hundred metres towards safety. On board Maria spotted her and yelled with excitement. 'It's Steph . . . she's made it!'

But Stephanie didn't make it. The young heroine, with all her colleagues safely on board, was within thirty metres of the shuttle when a shot rang out behind her, hitting her in the back, in the middle of the left side of the chest. The impact sent her crashing face first into the ground, the momentum of her running sending her skidding for another two metres. Within seconds a large red stain appeared around her lifeless young body. Like her gallant father so many years before and literally in another world she had been prepared to sacrifice herself for others. Those who could see out of the shuttle watched in horror as the blood poured from the front of her chest. The bullet had appeared to have ruptured her heart.

The willing hands by the hatch were to be left barren and before anyone could even comprehend what had happened, the hatch slammed shut automatically and the shuttle's engines roared to life. Carmel, ashen face, screamed, 'Stop it! For God's sake stop. Stop!'

But no one could stop the craft. Stephanie had seen to that. It started to gain speed and move away from their stricken colleague. The crew were stunned, shocked, but Carmel dissolved into complete hysteria at the loss of the person she most loved in her life. She screamed and fought in a manner which took nearly all of the others' efforts to restrain her. As the shuttle left the ground the power of her rage-cum-hysteria only worsened and she fought her colleagues as if she were fighting the perpetrator of the dreadful deed.

Maria began to fear for her crew's safety as Carmel's mayhem wreaked havoc.

'We'll be experiencing G forces soon,' she yelled, 'we must secure . . .' Her voice was drowned by ear-splitting shrieks. Loretta had managed to obtain a medical box, and was trying to open it, only to have it kicked from her grasp and the contents spilled everywhere. Whilst the others fought the wildcat, Kate retrieved a syringe and loaded an elephant-sized dose of sedative. She manouevred herself amongst the flailing arms and legs and copped a concussive blow in the face but, undaunted, she took aim and rammed the injection home, straight through Carmel's slacks into the upper part of her leg.

Carmel fought the paralysing effect of the drug, which gradually subdued her. Strange thoughts, bordering on hallucinations, took control of her mind. Memories of the happy childhood with her cheeky cousin, then the stark reality of the vile murder would reactivate bursts of hysteria, again requiring physical suppression by her colleagues. Eventually Carmel was controlled and confined. Her battered colleagues positioned themselves as well. The shuttle was a mess of littered equipment. Nevertheless, it continued its relentless journey back into space.

A similar, though less physical chaos had erupted on the space station. Put simply, nothing worked, except the very basics such as air supply. Even the back-ups could not be activated. Anderson might have won the mind game with Stephanie, but he had lost the battle. Now he would also lose his cool. He ejaculated useless and meaningless commands at his crew, none of whom could cope with the situation. One of his demands was for the DSP crew, but they were nowhere to be found.

They had managed to assemble amongst the chaos and hide and remain undetected, as all surveillance equipment had become inactive. Adam attempted to formulate a plan.

'I suspect that one of our members is responsible for this, so how do we get out?'

'I can get us to the dock,' replied Jack, 'but I don't know what Stephanie has in mind or whether it was Maria that set this off.'

'It was Stephanie,' interrupted Helen, 'I saw the transmission. She tried to bluff Anderson into allowing our release, but he wouldn't budge. Then she threatened him with shutting down the space station. But I don't think she had any choice then as I presume that she had preprogrammed the virus.'

'So whatever she planned has gone awry,' said Adam, 'at least in relation to our rescue, but what about the others? I wonder where they are?'

'If she planned to get us off, then I suspect that they are on their way back into space as well,' replied Jack. 'The point is that communications will eventually be restored, so there will only be a limited opportunity for us to escape.'

'Is there anything we can use to attempt a contact? I mean given that everything's wrecked on the space station.'

'We could program up an independent unit . . . with our own material,' said Helen, 'and communicate with the DSP.'

'Or the shuttle?' questioned Adam.

'Probably not if it is in flight,' said Jack. 'Also gaining

access to a unit without being spotted is probably impossible.'

'What about in the dock?' asked Alan. 'They have their own shuttles. I saw them when we arrived. If we could hide away in one of them, we could use their computer.'

'And hijack it?' asked Adam hopefully, but Jack shook his head. 'No . . . I suspect it would require an intact guidance system on the station, like ours does with the DSP, but I agree with Alan we could use it for communications.'

Having decided on a course of action, the group set off for the dock. It would require some stealth and diversion, during which several members of the space station crew would find themselves being suddenly overpowered and locked away in the most expedient chambers.

* * *

Back on the surface of the planet a gunman had sprinted down the runway after the escaping DSP shuttle, firing a few ineffectual shots. He then turned and walked back to the corpse on the ground. He roughly forced his toe under the body and flipped it over like the carcass of an animal, gasping at the grotesque sight of the almost totally bloodstained clothing. The chest area appeared shredded and there seemed to be blood-stained tissue projecting amongst the tattered clothing. He felt slightly sick at the inhuman sight but smiled as he congratulated himself on the accuracy of his shooting. An enormous pond of blood surrounded the body and had seeped up and covered the face and was now congealing in the hair. The perpetrator of the destruction grasped one of the feet and began to drag his prize towards the edge of the runway, anxious to display his booty to the colleagues he expected to follow. A deathly chill suddenly gripped him, however, as he heard a voice from behind.

'Hold it right there, and drop the gun!'

He turned slowly and, to his complete horror, discovered that the human remains that he was dragging had a gun drawn and aimed directly at his head.

'I said drop the gun . . . now!'

Unable to believe that anyone could exsanguinate and live, let alone hold someone at gunpoint, the man flinched slightly. This was sufficient to initiate an immediate response from the victim on the ground. Her gun roared to life and the man was struck on the cheek by a metal object which penetrated and lodged inside the roof of his mouth. He cried in pain and clasped his face, becoming entangled in a cord which issued from his cheek. With a cry of pain herself, Stephanie reached forward and grabbed the primitive-looking bolt action rifle which had been dropped like a hot potato. She quickly cocked it and, as the man turned his attention back to her, let fire a volley which struck her adversary in the groin. It flung him to the ground, where he writhed and yelped like a wounded dog.

The recoil of the rifle sent a mortifying searing pain through Stephanie's chest. So intense was it that she rapidly lost consciousness again. She was unaware of the figure who scrambled to her side and, as gently as he could, lifted her. Breaking into a run, he carried her to safety, whilst ignoring the screams for assistance from the gunman. The unbearable pain which had flung Stephanie into a coma now grabbed at her awareness as her porter's feet struck the ground and transmitted the vibration through her body.

Her eyesight blurred by pain, dirt and blood, she attempted to focus on her rescuer, and tried to utter her feelings. 'Help me . . . I'm shot . . . please . . . oh . . . I can't stand the pain . . .'

She shrieked and gasped, her respiration taking on a rapid shallow quality as every attempt to breathe seemed to tear her chest wide open. She was becalmed momentarily by a response from the person who held her.

'You'll be all right. Don't worry. Just try and hang on ... You'll be safe soon!'

'Leonard!' she said feebly, and to his amazement even managed a faint smile. However, Leonard doubted the validity of his reassurances as he noted the extent of Stephanie's blood loss. Blood still appeared to be seeping out of her chest, not to mention her suit, which was soaked, and there was an enormous pool left behind on the ground.

Coincidentally, as Stephanie drifted in and out of her semi-coma, only being awakened by the intensity of her pain, her cousin Carmel was undergoing a similar experience under the influence of the roughly administered sedative. As Leonard loaded his passenger, Stephanie once again uttered his name, but for the next part of the journey, tortured cries and gasping were all that she could manage. The pain of being moved again reactivated Stephanie's mind, but it was only momentary; a bright light shone in her face and she heard the sound of scissors hacking away her clothing. She couldn't see how many people attended her, though it seemed a few. She was aware of being naked and feeling deathly cold and heard loud exclamations:

"Her chest ... what has happened?"

She heard no more. An indeterminable time later she awoke, and on attempting to move, felt the searing pain in her chest return and a tug as if she were attached to something. She heard a voice whisper, 'She's awake!'

Stephanie wanted to move but didn't dare. She was in a smallish room. There were no windows that she could see. Her eyes focused on a person who was holding her hand. It was Mrs Hutchinson.

'I've been shot,' uttered Stephanie. Her comforter quickly reassured her. 'You're all right dear ... Don't worry ... You're safe.'

Another face appeared next to the motherly figure. It looked grim and concerned.

'Penny . . .' said Stephanie as she swam back to life.

'I thought you were dead,' said Penny in a matter of fact manner. 'You had blood everywhere. Mum's a nurse. She patched you up.'

'Do you have much pain?' asked Mrs Hutchinson.

'It's OK if I lie still,' replied Stephanie, 'and if I don't breathe too deeply.'

'I gave you some of my blood,' said Penny proudly. Stephanie's cheeky grin appeared. It immediately warmed the hearts of her saviours. Then she asked. 'Was it Leonard that saved me?'

'Yes. He actually saw you shot. The person that did it assumed you were dead and started to drag you away!'

'That's what brought me round,' said Stephanie, 'the pain nearly killed me!'

'Well,' continued Mrs Hitchinson, 'you shot the man with some sort of gun with a string attached. Then you grabbed his gun and shot him in the leg. Once he had been disarmed Leonard came and got you. He couldn't believe you had lost so much blood and survived.'

At that point she began laughing but managed to say, 'But we eventually found out why.'

As if she read Mrs Hutchinson's thoughts, Stephanie suddenly put her hands to her chest and exclaimed, 'My boobs!'

'Yes, your artificial breasts that were taped to your chest, I presume that they were filled with fluid.'

'Yes,' replied Stephanie, managing another grin, 'about two litres in each. I wanted to look impressive.'

'The bullet entered your back at an angle,' continued Mrs Hutchinson. 'It probably skated around the inside of a rib and came out the front. That's where it did most of the damage, It splintered the rib and lacerated the intercostal blood vessels, then ruptured the bags which were taped to your chest. You did lose a lot of blood, but when mixed with all the fluid it must have seemed like a torrent. When Leonard brought you back you can't imagine how terrible you looked.'

'Especially after how nice you looked before,' added Penny. Stephanie became more lucid by the minute. Now she was anxious. 'Oh my God! Sis . . . what will she think?'

'You have a sister!' exclaimed Penny.

'Actually she's a cousin. Carmel, you've met her. She'll think I'm dead, and so will the others. Where exactly are we?'

'You can't go anywhere at the moment, I'm afraid,' said Mrs Hutchinson. 'We're hidden . . . and besides to move you would be too painful.'

Stephanie managed a shallow sigh. Her plans appeared to have come unstuck. She had failed to secure the release of the crew members on the space station and she had probably devastated the rest by appearing to have been murdered. She voiced her regrets to her companions, who quickly reassured her. She was to discover that her actions had neutralised the forces in power for long enough to allow the opposition to mobilise. In fact communications were still out as a result of Stephanie's sabotage.

The three females chatted for the next two hours, Stephanie occasionally having to stop as a result of pain, whereupon her two eager attendants would hasten to her in an attempt to make her more comfortable. Eventually Leonard returned and beamed as he caught Stephanie's eye.

'Back from the grave, I see,' he remarked.

'Thanks to you,' replied Stephanie.

Leonard pulled up a chair and joined the other members of his family at the bedside. His mother cautioned him. 'We really should let her rest, we've been talking for ages.'

'No! Don't go,' protested Stephanie, 'it takes my mind off the pain. Please stay!'

Leonard gave his version of the rescue and some details about what had happened since Stephanie had set off the earlier chain of events. During a lull in the conversation, Mrs Hutchinson asked, 'How old are you Stephanie?'

'She won't answer that question,' laughed Leonard.

'Yes I will,' said Stephanie, contradicting him, 'I'm sixteen.'

Her attendants sat contemplating this fact for a minute. Then Mrs Hutchinson asked, 'By the way, Stephanie, what is that lump in your arm? Is it some sort of medical pellet?'

'It's a contraceptive pellet,' replied Stephanie, blushing as she noticed Leonard staring directly at her.

'Oh!' remarked Mrs Hutchinson, with a note of surprise or disapproval, Stephanie wasn't sure which, so she blurted out, 'But I'm still a virgin . . . I haven't needed it.'

'Why do you have it then?' said Penny, asking the obvious question.

'They're compulsory. Besides, it makes my boobs grow.'

Leonard steered the conversation away from its anatomical tilt. 'I'm surprised that someone as young as you was allowed to go on an interstellar mission.'

'It didn't start out as an interstellar mission,' replied Stephanie. 'Anyway you're right. Carmel and I both falsified our ages; the minimum age was supposed to be twenty-three.'

Stephanie began to feel weak and tired and Mrs Hutchinson insisted that she rest. Deep into the night she awoke to find that the lights were dimmed and that she was alone with Leonard. She smiled as she became aware of him, though she winced when she attempted to move. He took her right hand. She immediately drew it up to her right breast and she then applied his hand to the soft mound; she had developed considerably since the launch of the DSP and really no longer had any great need to augment her size. Having hardly appreciated the romance of being carried to safety by her gallant rescuer, she now intended to salvage some physical pleasure. It would be short-lived, however, as she soon drifted back to sleep again and would not re-awaken for several hours.

* * *

As the chaotic shuttle ride entered the upper atmosphere, Bud, who had tuned out from the crisis around him, had fought to crack Stephanie's security code and thus regain manual control of the shuttle. Sophisticated though the code was, Bud eventually achieved success and quickly announced to Maria, 'I've got it . . . we can take over and return if we want.'

Maria wasn't sure that she wanted to hear that news. Logic told her that there was nothing to be achieved by returning. After all, Stephanie had sacrificed her life so that they could escape. Why jeopardise it? Yet to leave the body of the person who had saved them on an alien planet seemed incomprehensible. Maria eventually passed judgement.

'The chances are that we would be shot up as well. If we're going to attempt heroics, let's head for the space station.'

'We'll have to orbit first,' replied Bud.

Maria nodded. She felt sick, as did the remainder of the shuttle crew, except for Carmel who was now deeply unconscious. Eventually they reached the familiar weightless environment of space and set about restoring order. The shuttle was somewhat cramped with the extra passengers, though it posed no particular technical problems. Maria and Bud planned to fill up any remaining space with the remainder of the crew. Bud probed the space station's defences and made a startling discovery.

'It's virtually shut down, and there are distress signals!'

Yvonne joined them and they all continued probing but no new information could be obtained.

'Try the DSP,' suggested Yvonne.

Bud flipped through a list of routine data, then exclaimed, 'There's a transmission coming into the DSP. And if I'm not mistaken . . .' Instead of finishing the sentence he flashed up a picture on the screen.

'Adam!' the three exclaimed together.

Adam responded immediately. 'I've got you. Where are you?'

'On the shuttle and orbiting,' replied Maria, 'we're making for the space station.'

'Good,' replied Adam, 'we are in the dock. We'll guide you in, the station's in chaos. Stephanie shut them down good an proper.'

No one responded, and Adam, sensing something was amiss, spoke again. 'Is everything OK?'

Maria replied in a halting voice. 'Adam . . . Stephanie was murdered. She didn't make it . . .'

Now it was Adam's turn to be silent, he eventually reappeared grim-faced.

'I read you . . . stand by.'

The shuttle continued its path towards the space station and docked completely unseen. Soon the remaining nineteen members of the crew were united and quickly pulled away in the direction of the DSP. As they docked, there wasn't a single member who didnt think of Stephanie; in fact they half expected the effervescent little imp to pop out and say, 'Surprise'. No such magic would be wrought, however, and the crew quickly manned their stations. They would find out soon after that they had escaped in the nick of time as the forces of evil, lead by Anderson, were on the point of cannibalising their craft and enslaving the crew completely.

The medical team, apart from battling their own melancholia, had to contend with profound depression amongst the crew, especially Carmel, though she tried hard not to let it influence her work. As they pulled away from the Proxima system, they analysed the voluminous data that Stephanie had pilfered. It drew them to some amazing conclusions, which Alex summed up.

'The absolute time scale exists all right, but the movement of the universe follows a helical path; we can either chase it, or hop across to the next loop, taking a short cut as it were.'

'What does it mean in practical terms?' asked Adam.

'It seems that we did some fairly daredevil manouevres without realising it previously. We need to take things more slowly and watch our maximum speed, especially in a craft this shape. Our best option is to take the short cut. It will mean a journey of six months, but it will mean that we return to our own system approximately six years after we left.'

'I think the shorter the journey the better,' said Adam, thinking seriously of the morale of his crew.

Whilst her colleagues headed for home, Stephanie recovered in the company of her new 'family'. However, all was not well on the planet. She had reached the stage of gentle ambulation when Mr Hutchinson approached her. His family stood at his side as he spoke.

'We have to move you, Stephanie. It's too dangerous for you to stay. We have to do it now whilst we still have the upper hand.'

'Where will you take me?'

Mr Hutchinson gave a wry smile as he answered, 'A long way from here . . . to safety.'

Mrs Hutchinson frowned, 'I don't think you're ready to travel, but we have no choice.'

Stephanie delivered her melting grin and replied, 'I'll be OK, don't worry!'

17

'Could I speak to Ben Andrews, please?'

'I'm afraid he isn't available, he's on duty tonight and still asleep,' replied Karen. 'May I ask who is calling?'

'Yes I'm sorry, I'm Peter Spence. I work with Ben . . .'

'Yes, of course,' interrupted Karen. 'Hang on, Peter, I'll just check . . .'

Karen deposited the telephone handset and went to check on her husband. She stole quietly into the darkened room, the thick curtains drawn and secured to keep out the bright afternoon sunshine. She watched Ben for a moment and wondered whether she should disturb him. He stirred in response to her presence and sat up.

'Oh! You're awake. I wasn't sure. Peter's on the phone.'

Ben leapt up, gave Karen a quick hug and hastened to the phone. 'Peter . . .'

'I'm sorry to disturb you, Ben, I just couldn't wait to tell you . . . I've sort of . . . worked something out.'

'Tell me!' said Ben.

'Well, I think that I have an explanation for the object that the astronomers saw.'

Ben went to sit down. Karen, who hovered in the background, provided a chair. She sensed something important and remained close by.

'Go on,' said Ben.

'It's to do with what the astronomers saw. You

remember how they saw the object which divided and part appeared to regress, but at each individual position was blue-shifted, which meant it should be travelling towards us. Well, the phenomenon would be explained if the object had been travelling in excess of the speed of light.'

Ben attempted to digest the scientific ramifications of Peter's theory. He concluded that it was feasible except for one reservation, which he voiced. 'But how can an object travel faster than the speed of light?'

'I don't know,' replied Peter, 'but I wouldn't be surprised if someone once said: How can anything travel faster than the speed of sound?'

Ben drew a long breath and replied, 'It's a very tempting explanation, Peter . . .'

'It also could mean that the DSP wasn't blown up after all,' interrupted Peter.

Ben was becoming more and more drawn in by Peter's theories and invited his young colleague to continue.

'How do you figure that?'

'It's possible that the explosion occurred behind the DSP and flung it forward. Remember we wondered about that? Well perhaps it has survived and is on its way back.'

'It's a tempting theory, Peter, but a bit hopeful, I'm afraid.'

'I guess so. I just had to tell someone. I'm sorry I disturbed you.'

'No . . . no . . . please don't apologise,' said Ben hastily, 'the super light speed theory would fit perfectly, as the actual object would be seen before the light from its previous positions reached us. You may have made a great discovery, though I'll be darned if I can see how it could happen. It would be interesting to get an update on what they can see at the observatory.'

'I've already done that,' came Peter's reply. 'They only have an image of one object now, still travelling towards us. They seem to have decided that it is just a comet and the previous phenomenon some sort of collision or partial disintegration. The interesting thing, though, is that it has already entered the boundary of our solar system.'

'In that case we may have some answers soon,' replied Ben.

The two then discussed some of the finer points of Peter's hypothesis and then ended the conversation. Ben recounted the details to Karen. She did not fully grasp the more technical points of the information but became excited nevertheless. The discussion was interrupted by another phone call which Karen answered.

A pause followed, then a polite female voice.

'Good afternoon. May I speak to Ben Andrews?'

'Who is calling, please?'

There was another pause, before the female spoke again. 'My name is Corinna Parker . . . it's about a scientific matter.'

Karen placed her hand over the telephone's mouthpiece and called to Ben.

'Do you want to speak to a Corinna Parker?'

'Never heard of her!' came Ben's reply. 'Can you ask her what she wants?'

'She already said it's about a scientific matter.'

'Wait a minute, I think she is a student,' muttered Ben, remembering the young woman whom he briefly encountered when he first met Peter. He sighed and walked to the phone again, grimacing as he approached.

'They're supposed to write to the director and obtain permission.'

However, having just received a reminder of what a youthful mind could achieve, he toned down his response.

'Hello, what can I do for you?'

'Hello, Mr Andrews,' said the polite voice, 'I am researching a report on a recently discovered comet, and a gentleman at the observatory seemed to think that you may have had some sort of communication from it.'

'Who are you exactly?'

'I'm a science student. I came to the communications centre recently, but it wasn't convenient to . . .'

'I'm sorry,' interrupted Ben, 'I can't help. You'll have to go through the director's office.'

Ben put down the receiver before the young woman could speak again and shook his head. Normally a patient individual, he 'apologised' beneath his breath.

'Sorry young lady . . . bad timing!'

Unable to return to sleep, Ben suggested an evening stroll with Karen, then dinner and before he knew it, he was at work and greeting Peter. They discussed Peter's theory again and again. Unfortunately the mysterious transmissions had come to an abrupt halt. In fact several weeks would pass before any new development would occur. During this time, there were a few more feelers from the press, but they were quickly dismissed. Then one night Ben received a note from the director. It stated that the director wished to show an individual around the department and that he would appreciate it if Ben or a colleague could be available. Ben decided that it would be a good opportunity for Peter to learn to deal with such situations and promptly delegated the task.

Ben wished Peter luck as he left. Approximately half an hour later the director, Rupert Gillespie, arrived with an attractive though determined-looking young woman, whom he introduced to Peter.

'Peter, this is Corinna Parker, she's researching a scientific project as part of her course.'

'We've already met,' announced Peter, looking pleasantly surprised and regretting that he had not taken advantage of the fact that he was already in possession of Corinna's phone number. He then studied her more closely. She looked different, more determined, yet particularly beautiful, even though she wore quite massive spectacles. She also wore a very fashionable suit-like outfit which included a short and seductively tight-fitting skirt. Rupert left the two alone and Peter soon found himself being interrogated unmercifully. It was as well that there were no state secrets to be revealed as the young man found his companion irresistable and would willingly have told her anything.

Fortunately, when she touched on the subject of the supposed comet, Peter managed to hold his tongue and plead ignorance. However, on recalling the conversation with Ben the following night, it seemed that she was more interested in technical aspects of the operations room itself and even wanted to learn about the more techncial aspects of the equipment. She also made copious notes and finally thanked Peter for his time.

'She sounds like quite a character,' remarked Ben later.

'She sure is . . . actually we've arranged to have lunch next week. She wants to show me her finished article.'

'What about that steady girlfriend, Peter?' asked Ben with a grin. 'You had better be careful!'

Peter laughed and replied, 'This Corinna bird is very attractive, but a bit too intense for me . . . it will be purely platonic!'

'Well, apologise to her for me. She rang me at home and I cut her a bit short . . . I was preoccupied with the DSP business.'

The two settled into their shift, mundane at first. It would become a night of nights. It happened as a déjà vu as Peter drew Ben's attention to the flashing call sign which returned for the first time for many weeks. They both turned and watched, fully expecting the usual disappointment to follow. However this time was different. After flashing for approximately two minutes, the image was replaced by a list of instructions and a programme directive.

Excitement gripped Ben and Peter. Ben quickly ran down the list and hastily commenced typing the programme, then, surprisingly, a list of questions appeared, personal questions, which took the form of dates mainly. Ben frowned as he typed them. Peter provided an explanation.

'It's some sort of security . . . so that only you can access the transmission.'

Ben nodded in agreement; he was too excited to think about it.

Then the screen lit up with Adam Coleman's image and the two spectators watched in awe.

'This is Captain Adam Coleman from the Deep Space Probe. We have not received replies from our previous transmissions to you. We expect to approach Earth in two weeks and will move into orbit. We await your instructions and send our good wishes.'

The screen went blank, the observers turned to each other and leapt to their feet, Ben giving a loud whoop and grasping Peter's hand and shaking it vigorously.

'Yeeeeah hoo . . . Peter . . . you were right! You little genius. Quick, the phone . . .'

Joe Sullivan found his slumber interrupted once again by an early morning call. This time he had no difficulty raising his level of consciousness as Ben screamed down the line. 'Joe . . . Joe . . . They're alive! They're alive! Adam has just spoken to us. It's fantastic!'

Joe made another early morning trek to the centre and was greeted by an absolutely ecstatic Ben, who recounted the events that had led to the reception of the transmission. Joe soon had the privilege of seeing the face of the man who had long been assumed dead and joined in the excitement, though a strange thought nagged at him. He would recount it later to his wife.

'There was something about Adam's expression. He

looked depressed.'

'That's not surprising after six years in space,' reassured Gloria.

'If only we'd received the earlier transmissions,' said Joe ruefully, 'but it shouldn't be too long before we can have two way conversations.'

'Are you going to release the information?'

'Not yet. I want to make absolutely sure that everything's all right. I couldn't stand the press having any reason to start another onslaught.'

However the press soon obtained another source of information in relation to the DSP in the form of the reception by a radio astronomy unit of the transmission sent by the crew as they had headed into the Proxima system. It received wide coverage for about three days. Then as nothing followed, the whole incident was widely criticised as a hoax. Joe maintained a steadfast no comment in response to those who tracked him down. The communications centre also came under seige with the result that Ben diverted transmissions from the DSP and hid them for later viewing.

No one linked the transmission from Proxima with the relentless approach of the 'comet'; news of which was very much relegated to the fine print of the newspapers. As the hubbub subsided, Ben retrieved the DSP transmissions. They had become highly technical, the crew obviously preparing for their expected arrival. Adam requested details of docking procedures and transport to Earth. He also questioned the lack of response from Earth. A conference between Joe, Ben and Peter mapped out a plan of action.

'Can we use the centre's transmitters to reply?' asked Joe.

'I'll have to ask Rupert,' replied Ben, 'which means letting the cat out of the bag.'

'I know what Rupert is like,' said Joe, 'although I hardly

know him personally, but I remember how he stuck up for us and how he offered employment to our scientists who got the bullet.'

'Me included,' added Ben with a grin, 'yes, I agree, with him behind us, all should go well.'

Joe and Ben arranged a meeting with the director the next day, whilst Peter kept a date with the vivacious Corinna. She proudly showed him her report .

'It's very impressive,' he remarked.

'I had a good instructor,' she replied and leant across and grasped his arm.

Peter responded with a somewhat gawky smile. He was quite besotted by this beautiful creature who, once again, was dressed quite seductively in a low cut summer frock. They completed their lunch and prepared to part company.

'I'd like to see you again,' said Corinna.

'That would be nice,' replied Peter awkwardly, '. . . er I have a girlfriend.'

Corinna laughed and replied, 'I promise to keep it strictly professional . . . give me a ring.'

She fluttered away with a wave. Peter, feeling quite flushed, contemplated a later rendezvous with his girlfriend. The relationship had very much stagnated and Corinna's overture didn't exactly help matters.

Joe, Ben and Rupert completed a successful meeting. Rupert was more than cooperative and promised the strictest confidence, though they all agreed that as the supposed comet approached and moved into orbit, they would break the news. They also agreed to prevent any sensitive details from being released prematurely, and they would instruct Adam to reduce his transmissions to those containing technical data only, as from now on, anything said by either party could be intercepted.

Having been stung by what they had thought was a false alarm, the media took a few days to pick up on the revelation regarding the reappearance of the DSP. However, once confirmed from other independant sources, the story dominated the news. Joe and his colleagues had steeled themselves for the attention that followed. They were ably supported by Rupert, everyone maintaining a stonewall 'no comment' and releasing only technical information about the arrival of the craft.

Nevertheless the media had no problems manufacturing their own versions of the phenomenon. Different newspapers enunciated their own emphasis: 'Miracle in space,' 'Return from black hole,' and even: 'Former Director vindicated,' screamed one headline, much to Joe's satisfaction.

Another point of safisfaction was Joe's eventual ability to converse with Adam, though it was tempered by the fact that it could be technical language only. Adam, still mystified about the paucity of response from Earth, could only assume that his earlier transmissions had provoked anxiety, perhaps in relation to the crisis on the Proxima Earth. He didn't realise that as yet these transmissions had never been deciphered.

With the abandonment of the interstellar space programme, facilities for retrieving the DSP crew were non-existent and they hastily prepared their own shuttle and contemplated another overcrowded ride, rather than fragment into smaller groups and use what was available. A long abandoned facility with an appropriate runway was reactivated and as the arrival approached, so did the euphoria.

To prevent a fiasco, personnel at the landing site were severely restricted to those who would operate the facility and immediate family members only. The crew would then be flown by conventional aircraft to a major airport where they could be seen by the press and general public. However, Joe insisted on taking Gloria, Karen and Millie. Ben, of course, would go and he in turn insisted on allowing

Peter to come. Peter, delighted at the opportunity, then asked if he could bring Corinna.

'What about that girlfriend of yours?' asked Ben doubtfully.

'Ex-girlfriend,' replied Peter, 'besides, Corinna has named me as a co author in her science article. I want to reward her.'

'Sure,' said Ben, 'how can I refuse a genius. Bring her along.'

In the end approximately 150 people formed the welcoming committee for the DSP crew. Corinna lost some of her charisma in Peter's eyes by not being ready when he called for her. However, she duly compensated with her stunning appearance. Her hair flowed freely instead of being caught up in the manner with which Peter was familiar. Her make-up accentuated every beautiful facial feature, especially her eyes, which on this occasion were unencumbered by the usual spectacles. She appeared breathless as she apologised.

'I'm sorry. I wanted to look my best.'

'You certainly look that,' he uttered, 'come on, let's go!'

As they drove to the landing area, Peter found himself looking frequently at the passenger's seat. Corinna sat very erect. Her short skirt had ridden up, revealing a pair of extremely seductive legs and her breasts thrust powerfully forward. She didn't say much, but she seemed excited and thanked Peter for his invitation.

'Thanks so much . . . isn't it exciting?'

'It sure is,' replied Peter, equally excited.

They approached a checkpoint and quickly dispensed with the formalities. There were still approximately two kilometres to the reception area.

'Look!' exclaimed Corinna suddenly, making Peter jump, 'it's them!'

Peter squinted, but it would be another couple of minutes

before he could make out the dot in the sky, which loomed larger by the minute. People were already assembled in a group to the side of the runway; some were already waving. A transport vehicle stood at the readiness to ferry the crew from the shuttle. As Peter and Corinna approached the building, she issued an instruction.

'Pull up here and go and join the others. I'll park the car.'

'But . . .'

'Go on. I made us late. I'll be right behind you!'

* * *

Maria had been given the honour of piloting the shuttle to Earth. Adam sat beside her. Carmel had been given the honour of being immediately behind, where Alex or Yvonne would normally have sat. Adam hoped that an early glimpse of Joe and his two daughters might compensate in some small way for the loss of Stephanie.

Maria brought the craft down to a perfect landing and it slipped past the centrally placed reception committee to the far end of the runway. She then turned it and commenced to taxi back to the group of welcomers. As it had minimal braking abilities, the shuttle had used up most of the length of the three kilometre runway. To Maria and Adam's surpise, they noted a car suddenly stop about 200 metres away and a young woman hastily leap out, leaving the driver's door wide open. She then hitched her already short skirt and kicked away a pair of high-heeled shoes and ran towards the shuttle, her blonde hair streaming behind her.

'Get a load of that!' exclaimed Maria, 'so much for the security around here.'

Ignoring the young woman, Maria completed her turn and commenced to taxi. Carmel peered over her shoulder and observed the figure who now chased them, waving wildly and obviously shouting, though her cries could not be heard. A horrible chill gripped Carmel as she relived Stephanie's last moments. Then . . . then . . .

'Stop! Stop! Oh Maria, stop! For God's sake . . . STOP!'

Maria's ears rung as Carmel screamed the final instruction. Neverthless the shuttle duly ground to a halt as Carmel delivered her next instruction.

'Open the hatch . . . I'm getting out!'

'But Carmel . . .' protested Maria.

'Let her go,' interrupted Adam, delighted at Carmel's elation on seeing whoever it was.

'Wait for me!' called back Carmel as she scrambled past her bewildered colleagues.

Maria peered out of the window. The young woman had almost reached the shuttle and was still waving in a frenzied manner. Carmel dropped from the hatch and ran towards her.

Meanwhile a blonde wig was plucked free and equally long and luxuriant rich brown tresses shaken loose. As the two females approached on a relentless collision course, one commenced sobbing, the other screeched like a mad person.

'Sis . . . oh Sis . . . at last!'

Carmel and Stephanie embraced with such force that both would retain the bruises for days. As Carmel sobbed uncontrollably on her resurrected cousin, the latter looked up, and releasing an arm, waved wildly to the dot-like figures in the cockpit of the shuttle.

Maria stared unbelievingly at what she could just make out as the cheeky grin that had been so indelibly imprinted on her mind. She leapt from her seat and screamed. 'It's Stephanie'. Amazed at the lack of response, this time she roared, 'ITS STEPHANIE! What's the matter, are you deaf?'

Those nearest the hatch responded and within a few seconds the re-united cousins were being hauled in, as pandemonium broke out.

Only Loretta managed a sober comment to Kate before they joined the mêlée. 'OK, you tell me. How did she do that?'

Maria was at a loss as to whether to join in the fracas or respond to the pleadings from the tower. Adam pushed her away into the depths of the shuttle.

'Go on, join in, I'll take us in!'

Carmel's hysteria came close to matching the level it had reached when she thought that her beloved had been snatched for eternity. This time no one cared, in fact many joined in.

'Sorry about the delay,' said Adam to the bewildered tower staff, 'we . . . er . . . had to pick up a passenger.'

As a security vehicle reached the abandoned car, the shuttle commenced taxiing once more and eventually settled at its correct point of destination. Soon a wildly excited, laughing, tearstained group of space travellers spilled from the shuttle. They declined the transport and instead half skipped towards the terminal.

Peter had joined Ben and Joe and Joe's family. Puzzled by the delay at the end of the runway, which was really too far away for them to see, they now watched the euphoric crew approach. Chaired high above the group was a young woman with her skirt roughly pulled above her waist and supported by a myriad of hands.

'Corinna!' exclaimed Peter in amazement.

'Stephanie!' squealed Karen and Millie. '. . . and Carmel!'

As relatives surged forwards, the DSP crew fragmented and Stephanie was deposited on the ground. Carmel held her arm in a vice-like grip as they approached their 'family.'

'Uncle Joe,' yelled Stephanie, as she spotted the group.

To Joe and his family Carmel and Stephanie made an incongruous pair. Carmel's face was red raw from crying. She seemed emotionally drained and would be unable to speak without bursting back into tears and clasping Stephanie. The latter, on the other hand, seemed elated, smartly dressed in contrast to the 'uniforms' worn by the remainder of the crew, though her previously perfect make-up was smeared as a result of a thousand kisses and embraces. In amongst the wild reunion, Stephanie managed to release an arm and draw in Peter.

'I'm sorry about the deception Peter, I'm Stephanie!'

She then reached out and kissed the bewildered young man, depositing the remains of her smudged lipstick on his mouth.

Totally incoherent conversations filled the air as the DSP crew struggled to cope with the dual excitement of returning home and being reunited with their heroine, whose 'death' had turned their return journey into a melancholic nightmare. Whilst the crew attempted to reunite with their families, they desperately longed to hear the mechanism of Stephanie's return from the grave, not to mention her seemingly impossible feat of returning home before them.

18

The now complete twenty member crew of the DSP had been sequestered at Adam's request. Stephanie's miraculous reappearance had charged an emotional bomb in what had been a void of depression. She now addressed her colleagues in an attempt to defuse the situation. Carmel sat glued to her, more like a conjoined twin than a cousin.

'All the blood that you saw, was blood-stained fluid from my plastic boobs,' said Stephanie, 'though I was hurt pretty badly. I managed to shoot the swine in the face with a line gun, then grab his gun and fire into his leg. The recoil made me feel as if I was split in two and I went out like a light again. Penny's brother rescued me. Their mother is a nurse and she patched me up . . . Penny even gave me some blood, as she was the only one compatible, though she's too small to give much.'

'You were very lucky,' said Anna.

'I'll say. I was a mess. Every tiny movement hurt like crazy. Anyway the Hutchinsons, that's Penny's family, told me that I had to escape and the only hope was whilst the communications were knocked out. They took me to an interstellar craft. It was round and saucer-shaped, just like we predicted. They leave from the ground. In fact the space station's a bit of a relic, it's been taken over by Anderson for military purposes. The journey was hellish, I've never ever felt pain like it, I could feel the splintered rib gouging into me.' She gave a slight shudder in response to the recollection.

'They gave me a crash course in operating the saucer, though it's very straightforward and all automatic; you just dial up where you want to go and when. You then get a list of options and off you go! It was identical with the programme that I stole and loaded into the shuttle computer . . . I hoped that you would find it and use it.'

'We did,' said Adam, 'but how did you know what time we would choose?'

'I assumed that you would take the short cut,' replied Stephanie. 'It was the safest for the DSP, even though it meant arriving back in six years, Earth time, I presumed that the six month journey would be most appealing.'

'It was the most dreadful six months of our lives,' said Maria, 'without you.'

'My journey was no picnic either,' continued Stephanie, 'you've no idea what six months in a sardine can is like . . . or at least five months.'

'Who came with you?' asked Adam.

Stephanie grimaced and replied, 'That's the point. No one came! It was gruesome, like solitary confinement. I was so ill at first, I didn't care. I developed an infection in the gunshot wound and I thought I would die. That helped to pass about six weeks. I was delirious most of the time. But then I recovered. It was worse, I even ended up talking to myself. However I occupied myself by analysing all the equipment on the saucer and studying the interstellar mechanics. Wait until you see it!'

'Where is the saucer?' asked Yvonne.

'Hidden in a rain forest in Queensland, Australia. It's brilliant to land. You can just glide around and park it under a tree. It took me a week to get back to civilisation and then back here; I arrived about five weeks ago. I assumed that the whole world would know that the DSP was coming, so I became worried when there was no news. I looked up the old newspapers from when we disappeared. They thought we were blown up all right. Everyone in the programme copped the blame and were fired.'

'Just as we thought,' said Alex.

'Exactly, so I didn't know what to do. I thought that if I went to Uncle Joe that I might cause more trouble for him, especially if I was exposed as a dizzy teenager who had dreamed up some far-fetched hoax. Apart from that I didn't want to reveal the saucer, so it was dress up time again. I didn't know where to look at first, but then I found a report about a strange comet. That led me to an observatory, then to a communications centre. Lo and behold, Ben Andrews worked there. I managed to bluff my way in and start loading the recognition code for the DSP, but I didn't have time to complete it. Ben appeared, but he didn't recognise me. Then, when I tried to ring him he fobbed me off, so I ended up approaching the director, but it took several weeks to get back in. All the reception codes had been scrapped, so I managed to slip in a programme whilst this nice young guy, Peter, was showing me around. Then ... bingo ... you were on the air! Everything was still very secretive, though, so I thought it safest if I kept a low profile, until today. I wasn't going to miss the homecoming for anything, though I guess we'll have some explaining to do.'

'Yes indeed,' said Adam, 'we can't disguise the fact that you were already here.'

'I'd planned to wait in orbit until you arrived, but when there was no sign of you, I was going nuts after five months ...'

'This has been much more exciting,' said Maria.

'Well ... we'd better return to the throng outside,' said Adam. 'Thanks, Steph. We'll never forget this day.'

Later that day Carmel and Stephanie attempted to relax

with Joe and his family.

'Everyone has grown up,' remarked Stephanie, looking particularly at Millie who, at nineteen, was now biologically older than herself.

'I can't comprehend that you have only been away for barely two years,' replied Millie, 'though you look more mature, Steph.'

'You should have seen her six months ago, dressed up as a thirteen year old,' said Carmel with a laugh.

In spite of the day's excitement, the now scattered DSP crew would retire early that night, though Carmel, who insisted on sleeping in the same room as Stephanie, chatted idly.

'We did it, Sis . . . Pity you had to scare me to death, though!'

'I'm sorry,' replied Stephanie, '. . . yes, it was great . . . except for one thing.'

'What's that?'

'I fell in love . . . with Penny's brother . . . I even had him alone at one stage!'

'So what happened?'

'Nothing! Unfortunately it was after I'd been shot. I was in too much damned pain.'

They both laughed at the unfortunate situation, then Stephanie continued, 'So after all the adventures . . . I'm still a virgin!'

'Go to sleep! . . . You brat!'

The following morning Peter paid an unexpected visit to the Sullivan household. Stephanie greeted him warmly and they spent about half an hour chatting in the garden, then Stephanie announced: 'Peter's going to give me a lift back to my flat to pick up a few clothes.'

They hurried past a few photographers and were soon underway. Stephanie wore the same outfit, as it was the only one she had with her. Re-installed in the front passenger seat of Peter's car, she presented the same seductive picture as that of the day before. They eventually alighted from the car, whereupon Stephanie took Peter's arm and pressed her breast close as they walked to the door. Once inside, she detached herself and said, 'I'll just go and change. Come and talk to me.'

Peter obeyed and she took his hand and led him to the bedroom. She then slid down her skirt, placed it over a chair and peeled off her tights, turning her back slightly to reveal her near naked buttocks, decorated only by a tiny pair of panties.

'I'll show you where I was shot,' said Stephanie and turned to face Peter. As she did so, she unbuttoned her blouse and removed her bra. She approached him and stood directly in front of him. She then placed his hand on her left breast and made him cup it whilst she pointed to the scar.

'It was very painful,' she whispered.

Peter stood, unable to speak, though very aroused. Stephanie then removed his hand and turned her back and whispered again, 'Can you see where the bullet went in?'

'Yes!'

She backed against him and drew his arms around her, placing both hands on her breasts for a minute. She then turned and kissed him passionately and spoke softly.

'Did you make love to your girlfriend?'

'Yes . . . I did!'

'Then take off your clothes and show me how!' said Stephanie nervously.

'OK . . .' The mesmerised Peter obeyed.

As he obliged, Stephanie slid away the last brief string that barely protected her fragile virginity. Within minutes she would be conquered. Or was it she who conquered? One never knew with Stephanie.

And so the passions that had first been lit so many

millions of miles away were finally fully ignited and satisfied and the child was bid farewell. The mistress of disguise would return to the land of the origins of her womanly awakenings; once again she would shatter light and time to go beyond the barrier in her triumphant return to Proxima.